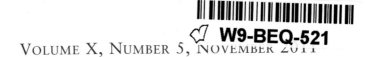

VOLUME X, NUMBER 5, NOVEMBER 2011

CLINICAL UPDATES IN WOMEN'S HEALTH CARE

Pain Management

Andrea J. Rapkin, MD
Department of Obstetrics
and Gynecology
David Geffen School of
Medicine at University of
California, Los Angeles
Los Angeles, California

Tamara G. Hartshorn, MD
Department of Obstetrics
and Gynecology
David Geffen School of
Medicine at University of
California, Los Angeles
Los Angeles, California

Parisa Partownavid, MD
Department of Anesthesiology
David Geffen School of
Medicine at University of
California, Los Angeles
Los Angeles, California

THE AMERICAN COLLEGE OF
OBSTETRICIANS AND GYNECOLOGISTS
Women's Health Care Physicians

Online access for subscribers—www.clinicalupdates.org

Clinical Updates in Women's Health Care is published quarterly by the American College of Obstetricians and Gynecologists (the College). This series represents the knowledge and experience of the authors and does not necessarily reflect the policy of the American College of Obstetricians and Gynecologists. The recommendations do not dictate an exclusive course of treatment or of practice. Variations taking into account the needs of the individual patient, resources, and limitations unique to the institution or type of practice may be appropriate.

Editorial Office:
130 Nickerson Street, Suite 211
Seattle, Washington 98109-1658

ISSN: 1536-3619
ISBN: 978-1-934984-09-3

12345/54321

CU048

Contents

After reading *Pain Management,* go to
www.clinicalupdates.org

- Complete and submit the CME questions online—automatically add 5 CME credits to your College cognate transcript. CME credit is available for all titles posted online.
- View links to resources related to pain management.
  — American Pain Society
    www.ampainsoc.org
  — American Academy of Pain Management
    www.aapainmanage.org
  — International Pelvic Pain Society
    www.pelvicpain.org
  — International Association for the Study of Pain
    www.iasp-pain.org
  — National Vulvodynia Association
    www.nva.org
- Order College patient education material.
- See full text of past issues and any relevant changes or updates.

Continuing Medical Education

Objectives

This monograph is designed to enable obstetrician–gynecologists to do the following:

- Understand the basis for acute and chronic pain
- Counsel patients about lifestyle modifications to decrease the risk of pain
- Identify the pathophysiology and underlying causes of pain
- Monitor risk factors and screen patients accordingly
- Understand the mechanisms of pharmacologic alleviation of pain
- Evaluate and treat patients with pharmacologic and nonpharmacologic therapies
- Understand the complications associated with pain management
- Make appropriate referrals of patients with complicated conditions

ACCME Accreditation

The American College of Obstetricians and Gynecologists is accredited by the Accreditation Council for Continuing Medical Education (ACCME) to provide continuing medical education for physicians.

AMA PRA Category 1 Credit™ and College Cognate Credit

The American College of Obstetricians and Gynecologists designates this educational activity for a maximum of 5 AMA PRA Category 1 Credit(s)™ or up to a maximum of 5 Category 1 College Cognate Credit(s). Physicians should only claim credit commensurate with the extent of their participation in the activity.

Credit for *Clinical Updates in Women's Health Care: Pain Management*, Volume X, Number 5, November 2011, is initially available through December 2014. During that year, the unit will be re-evaluated. If the content remains current, credit is extended for an additional 3 years.

Disclosure Statement

Current guidelines state that continuing medical education (CME) providers must ensure that CME activities are free from the control of any commercial interest. All authors, editorial board members, and reviewers declare that neither they nor any business associate nor any member of their immediate families has material interest, financial interest, or other relationships with any company manufacturing commercial products relative to the topics included in this publication or with any provider of commercial services discussed in this publication except for Morton Stenchever, MD, who has financial interests in Merck, Pfizer, Bristol Myers, GlaxoSmithKline, and Amgen; Raul Artal, MD, who has been involved with clinical trials with Nascent, Solvay, Xenodyne, Symbollon Pharmaceuticals, and Columbia Laboratories; and Julia Schlam Edelman, MD, who has financial interests in Alnylam Pharmaceuticals and Intelligent Bio-Systems. Any conflicts have been resolved through group and outside review of all content.

See page vi for submission of CME credits.

Foreword

Pain is one of the most common symptoms for which women consult their physicians. The pain may be acute, which requires immediate diagnosis and treatment of the cause; it may be chronic in nature, which requires careful evaluation; or it may be a multifactorial problem, which requires involvement of a team of specialists. The reasons for pain symptoms in patients who visit their obstetrician–gynecologists are many and varied and, at times, challenging to understand. This monograph, prepared by experts in pain management, should be of great value to obstetrician–gynecologists in providing care to patients who are experiencing a variety of conditions. The authors address the diagnosis and management of most of the obstetric–gynecologic conditions that can cause pain. Treatment options are discussed in detail, and emphasis is placed on improving the quality of life for such patients. Relieving pain associated with some conditions is not always possible, but the authors offer strategies for decreasing the stress of chronic pain that these patients often experience.

Morton A. Stenchever, MD
Editor

ABSTRACT. *Pelvic pain is one of the most common problems treated by the obstetrician–gynecologist. Chronic pelvic pain and pain related to the perioperative period, pregnancy, and terminal illness all present unique challenges. Chronic pain states are maintained by neuroplastic alterations in the modulation and perception of sensory signaling in the spinal cord and brain. As a result of these changes in neural processing, the pain experienced by the affected patient is out of proportion to the visualized pathology. Women with chronic pelvic pain often have symptoms that are derived from more than one pelvic visceral and somatic structure. Endometriosis, bladder pain syndrome, and irritable bowel syndrome are the most common visceral sources of chronic pelvic pain. Myofascial pain and neuropathic pain of the pelvic floor and abdominal wall are very prevalent and typically remain unrecognized. Patients with psychologic symptoms, such as anxiety and depression, can maintain the feelings of helplessness and hopelessness associated with chronic pelvic pain and this must be addressed. The current conceptualization of chronic pelvic pain reflects the biopsychosocial basis of the symptoms and successful treatment often requires multidisciplinary management. The multidisciplinary team comprises the obstetrician–gynecologist and when indicated, other subspecialists, such as urologists, gastroenterologists, anesthesiologists, and psychiatrists. Psychologists are important for the management of anxiety, depression, and stress. Physical therapists are needed for the treatment of myofascial pain. Pharmacotherapy includes hormonal suppression for pain related to the menstrual cycle and antidepressants, anticonvulsants, and local anesthetics to down-regulate nerve firing thresholds and improve mood. Surgery can be highly effective for some gynecologic pain disorders, such as endometriosis. The goal is by necessity, not always to achieve a pain-free state but to aim for an improved quality of life, optimal* *mood and sexual functioning, and a shift from "small life, large pain" to "large life, small pain."*

Comanagement with anesthesiologists also is crucial in the perioperative period. Postoperative pain control aims to reduce pain at the central level, decrease local inflammation, and decrease the incidence of adverse postoperative outcomes. Appropriate selection of specific pharmacologic agents, knowledge of safe dosage range, and novel routes of administration can increase the patient's functional and psychologic well-being, shorten her hospital stay, and reduce costs.

Pregnancy can present special challenges for pain management. Pain that occurs during pregnancy can be related to a preexisting chronic pelvic pain condition or may emerge as a new problem during the course of the pregnancy. In both situations, teratogenic medications must be avoided and the fetus protected. Labor and delivery also are painful and require judicious use of analgesic agents or, in the case of surgical delivery, anesthesia.

Optimal pain management for women with terminal illness must address not only the pain, but also anxiety, depression, agitation, weakness, nausea, loss of appetite, and poor sleep in an effort to improve the ability to cope with therapy and the quality of daily life.

Although likely underreported, an estimated 12–15% of women have signs or symptoms of chronic pelvic pain (1). More specifically, prevalence estimates for dyspareunia range from as low as 3% to as high as 43% depending on the age, culture, and method of obtaining the information (2). Chronic pelvic pain is the indication for approximately 10% of gynecologic referrals, up to 45% of laparoscopic evaluations, and at least 20% of hysterectomies performed in the United States (3). It often is associated with depression, anxiety, and other mood disorders (4). The combination of physical and emotional disorders and disability has a major effect on society and accounts for significant indirect costs, with up to a 45% reduction in work productivity and a 15% increase in time lost from work (1).

Obstetrician–gynecologists play a crucial role in the management of pelvic pain in women because they frequently are the first specialists consulted for pelvic pain problems. The basic science, epidemiology, differential diagnosis, and condition-specific and multidisciplinary management of chronic pain in women are outlined in this monograph. The most effective management strategies for chronic pelvic pain are multidisciplinary and can involve the use of pharmacotherapy, surgery, psychology, physical therapy, and complementary and alternative medicine (CAM) approaches, all of which are discussed. Additionally, the management strategies for postoperative pain, pregnancy-related pain, and pain related to terminal illness are addressed. A brief review of the pharmacology and therapeutics of medications used to treat chronic pelvic pain and perioperative pain, such as hormonal agents, anticonvulsants, antidepressants, local anesthetics, narcotics and nonsteroidal antiinflammatory drugs (NSAIDs) is included. Also discussed are the special considerations for management of pelvic pain in pregnant women, older women, and patients with narcotic addiction or tolerance.

Basic Science Update

Pain can be conceptualized as nociceptive, inflammatory, or neuropathic. Nociceptive pain is caused by stimulation of peripheral nerve fibers that respond only to stimuli approaching or exceeding harmful intensity (nociceptors). Most nociceptors are found in the skin or the walls of viscera. Mechanisms of visceral pain are explained in the following section "Neural Circuitry."

Inflammation occurs after tissue injury and involves the release of many chemicals, the most important of which may be prostaglandins (PGs). Prostaglandin release and induction of the enzyme involved in PG formation, cyclooxygenase-2 (COX-2), in the dorsal horn neurons are important in the generation of inflammatory pain hypersensitivity. Prostaglandins are used in the pharmacologic management of chronic pain states that involve inflammation, such as dysmenorrhea, endometriosis, and postoperative pain.

Damage to a peripheral nerve leads to subsequent changes in the spinal cord and brain and can result in neuropathic pain. Stimuli to the nerve in this setting produce a much greater magnitude of response than after an inflammatory stimulus that does not involve peripheral nerve damage (5). It is notable that the pharmacologic agents most useful in treating neuropathic pain affect sodium or calcium channel chemistry. Chronic pain associated with central sensitization and "plastic" changes in the central nervous system (CNS) also are considered to be a form of neuropathic pain.

Neural Circuitry

A thorough understanding of the neuroanatomy of the visceral and somatic pelvic structures is imperative for clinical evaluation of women with pelvic pain. Current information regarding mechanisms of neural signaling in the CNS (spinal cord and brain) also are presented to clarify how an acute stimulus or pain can transition into a chronic pain state.

The complexity and overlapping nature of the pelvic neurophysiology lends itself to interactions between the visceral and somatic nervous systems as well as between the reproductive, gastrointestinal (GI), and urinary systems (Fig. 1 [see color plate]) (6). Pelvic structures have a dual innervation by way of the somatic sensory and autonomic nervous systems.

Pelvic pain can derive from the viscera alone (uterus, adnexae, intestine, urinary tract, and visceral peritoneum) as a purely visceral pain or, more typically, include a component of referred visceral pain. True visceral pain is a diffuse, poorly localized sensation. Referred visceral pain is perceived to emanate from overlying somatic tissues that share dermatomal innervation with the involved viscera. Referred pain is a sharper and more localized pain than true visceral pain. Referred visceral pain is not accompanied by neurovegetative signs. The upper vagina, cervix, uterus, and adnexae share common visceral innervations with the large intestine, rectum, bladder, lower ureters, and lower small intestine (Fig. 1 [see color plate], Fig. 2 [see color plate], and Table 1). Therefore, pain from the reproductive organs, genitourinary (GU) tract, and GI tract is referred to the same dermatomes.

The pelvic organs are innervated by thoracolumbar and sacral autonomic nerves as well as the lumbosacral somatic sensory nerves that supply the overlying somatic structures, eg, abdominal wall, lower back, pelvic floor, vagina, vulva, urethra, rectum, and perineum.

Table 1. Innervation of the Pelvic Organs and Surrounding Somatic Tissues

Anatomic Structure	Spinal Segments	Nerves
Rectosigmoid, rectum and internal anal sphincter, upper vagina, cervix, lower uterine segment, uterosacral and cardinal ligaments, lower ureters, posterior urethra, and bladder trigone	S-2–S-4	Pelvic (sacral) autonomics (parasympathetics)
Terminal ileum, cecum, appendix, distal large bowel, upper bladder uterine fundus, broad ligament, and proximal fallopian tubes	T-11–T-12 and L-1	Thoracolumbar autonomics (sympathetics) through the inferior hypogastric plexus
Ascending colon, transverse colon, and descending colon	S-2–S-4	Pelvic autonomics through the inferior hypogastric plexus
	L-1–L-2	Lumbar autonomics through celiac, mesenteric, and superior hypogastric plexuses
Outer two thirds of fallopian tubes and upper ureters	T-9–T-10	Thoracic autonomics through aortic and superior mesenteric plexuses
Ovaries	T-9–T-10	Thoracic autonomics through renal and aortic plexuses and celiac and mesenteric ganglia
Lower abdominal wall and inguinal region	T-12–L-1	Iliohypogastric nerve
	T-12–L-1	Ilioinguinal nerve
	L-1–L-2	Genitofemoral nerve
External anal sphincter and puborectalis muscle	S-2–S-4	Medial branches of the pudendal nerve
Perineum, vulva, and lower vagina	S-2–S-4, L-1, and L-2	Pudendal nerve, vaginal branch of S-2, ilioinguinal nerve, genital branch of genitofemoral nerve, and posterofemoral cutaneous nerve
Pelvic floor muscles, levator ani muscles (puborectalis, iliococcygeus, and piriformis), and obturator internus	S-2–S-4	Pudendal nerve and division of sacral nerves (S-2–S-3) mingled with fibers of the inferior hypogastric plexus

The pelvic viscera, visceral peritoneum, and vasculature are innervated by corresponding afferent and efferent autonomic branches. The inferior hypogastric plexus is the major autonomic center that subserves painful sensations from the midline pelvic organs. Noxious stimuli from the pelvis are transmitted by at least five pathways, three of which pass through the inferior hypogastric plexus. The inferior hypogastric plexus originates from thoracic and lumbar spinal segments (T-11 through T-12) and gives rise to three other plexuses: 1) rectal, 2) uterovaginal, and 3) vesical. Corresponding afferent (sensory) branches are activated in response to noxious stimuli, such as distention, ischemia, or spasm.

The afferent innervation of the upper vagina, cervix, uterus, proximal fallopian tubes, upper bladder, and ascending, transverse, and sigmoid colon are derived from T-10–L-1 spinal segments (Table 1). More specifically, impulses from these structures travel with the thoracolumbar autonomics through the inferior hypogastric plexus to the hypogastric nerve, then to the superior hypogastric plexus, and finally to the lower thoracic and lumbar nerves, entering the spinal cord at segments T-10 through L-1. The distal fallopian tube, ovary, and upper ureter are innervated by sympathetic nerves traveling with the ovarian vessels, entering the spinal cord at segments T-9 through T-10, and as such, they bypass the superior and inferior hypogastric plexes.

The sacral plexus (S-2–S-4) provides the sacral autonomic innervation to the upper vagina, cervix, uterus, the bladder, lower ureters, and rectosigmoid by way of the pelvic splanchnic nerves. The vagina, vulva, perineum and anus, and pelvic floor muscles are innervated by the pudendal nerve by way of S-2–S-4 nerves that mingle with fibers from the inferior hypogastric plexus. The efferent branches are the motor component of the system and include the sympathetic (T-10–L-2) and parasympathetic (S-2–S-4) nerve fibers that supply the pelvic organs. Innervation of the abdominal wall is derived from the spinal nerves (T-10–L-2), primarily through the iliohypogastric and ilioinguinal nerves (T-12–L-2) and the genitofemoral nerve (L-1–L-2) (Fig. 3).

Evolutionarily, pain serves an important purpose as a warning system. After an injury, the release of inflammatory chemicals cause hyperactivity of the pain system from the dorsal horn of the spinal cord to the brain.

Peripheral and Central Sensitization

Peripheral sensitization occurs after any inflammatory insult, such as infection, surgery, or injury, and results in reduced amplitude and increased responsiveness of the pain receptors

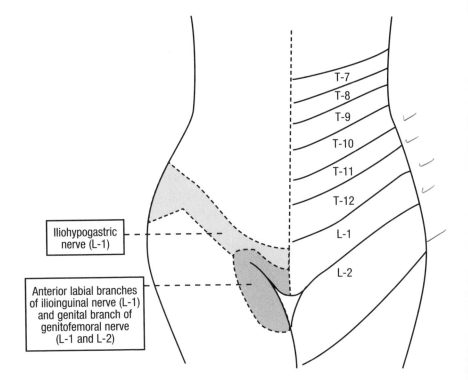

Fig. 3. Cutaneous innervations and dermatomes of the anterior abdominal wall.

(nociceptors) in the damaged tissue. It resolves with healing. In contrast, central sensitization involves a wide range of functional, chemical, and structural changes in neural processing (5). With central sensitization, alterations in CNS processing change how the brain responds to afferent input. This change in CNS processing reflects a malleability (as opposed to a hard wired system) that is called *neural plasticity*. With tissue injury, the noxious stimuli are transmitted by A delta fibers and C fibers, including a subset of C fibers called "silent" afferents that usually are not activated. A large proportion of visceral afferents from the viscera is of the silent type. Once these are activated, the dorsal horn of the spinal cord is flooded with noxious chemical stimuli that over time can lead to upregulation of the signaling in the dorsal horn and brain, and pain sensitivity remains amplified, even in the absence of peripheral pathology.

Allodynia
Hyperalgesia

With this process of central sensitization, the threshold for activation of the second-order neurons in the spinal cord decreases and the physiologic response to subsequent stimuli is altered. Allodynia and hyperalgesia ensue, whereby normally innocuous stimuli now result in painful sensation (allodynia) and moderately discomforting noxious stimuli are now perceived to be more intense (hyperalgesia) and are felt over a larger receptive field.

After central sensitization has occurred, the dorsal horn neurons manifest a number of electrophysiologic changes, including the development of spontaneous activity, enlarged receptive fields, and a lowered threshold for firing. Central sensitization involves increased membrane excitability, more efficient synaptic connectivity, and reduced central inhibition. Impulses that previously would not have reached the threshold are now facilitated and amplified. In chronic pain states, the pain is no longer adaptive, and the initial painful input produces a persistent "abnormal state of hyperresponsiveness characterized by increased gain of the nociceptive system" (5). It is not known why in some individuals or in certain settings, prolonged stimuli or injury will result in sensitization.

The chemistry underlying the triggering and maintenance of this altered functional state is complex and an area of active research. The continued exposure to noxious stimuli results in three phenomena: 1) changes in the threshold and activation of these postsynaptic spinal cord receptors, 2) increase in the inward current through ion channels, 3) altered activity of many chemicals, including γ-aminobutyric acid (GABA) and glycine, which leads to a reduction in the threshold for activation by peripheral stimuli. Neurons begin to respond to both innocuous and noxious stimuli in the same manner (5). Ultimately, long-term pain memory, called long-term potentiation, is established.

Changes in the Brain

Chronic pain has been associated with changes in cortical volume and cortical reorganization (7). Review of more than 100 brain imaging studies concluded that brain signaling patterns in patients with clinical pain syndromes differ from those in normal patients in response to the same stimulus. There is no one pain center in the brain; pain can be perceived if a number of cortical structures are stimulated even without neural input from the periphery. Results from functional magnetic resonance imaging (MRI) and positron emission tomography studies during acute and chronic pain states affirm changes in various brain structures. Specifically, the anterior cingulate cortex and insula are parts of the limbic system and serve in part to determine the emotional or affective dimension of pain. The prefrontal cortex is thought to encode the cognitive aspects of pain, including the meaning of the pain and coping with pain, and may modulate in a "top down" fashion, the signaling in the periaqueductal gray region in the brainstem to decrease pain (7). The discussion on how to recognize an acute pain state from exacerbation of a chronic pain state in a clinical setting is given in the section "Diagnosis."

Pelvic Organ Interconnections

Neural interconnections between viscera, also known as cross-talk, are another source of neuromodulation important to the understanding of chronic pelvic pain. As noted earlier, noxious stimuli travel from the viscera to the spinal cord by way of A delta fibers and C fibers. Within the dorsal root ganglia and the spinal cord, these converge with and have the ability to stimulate adjacent unmyelinated nerves from other uninvolved organs. The end effect is the lowered threshold for response from an organ that is not directly involved (8). The visceral fibers also converge on second-order neurons that receive input from somatic tissues, such as muscle and subcutaneous tissue in same neurotome. This viscerovisceral or viscerosomatic convergence within the spinal cord primarily is caused by the shared neural pathways of the pelvic organs and by the overlying somatic structures. Cross-sensitization implies that dysfunction or irritation in one pelvic organ decreases the threshold for sensation in a nearby structure as a result of inflammation, neural upregulation, or both.

Mediators of Pain

PROSTAGLANDINS

Prostaglandins (named so, because they were originally believed to be produced in the prostate) are structures derived from unsaturated 20-carbon fatty acids, primarily arachidonic acid, through the cyclooxygenase or the lipoxygenase pathway. They are potent mediators of many physiologic processes, including pain. The role of PGs in inflammatory and nociceptive processes is not completely understood, but they are believed to sensitize the spinal neurons to pain and induce contraction or relaxation of the smooth muscle in different organ systems, thus producing adverse effects (uterine cramps, nausea, vomiting, or diarrhea).

Prostaglandin production is catalyzed by two different iso-enzymes: 1) cyclooxygenase-1 (COX-1) and 2) COX-2 (Fig. 4). The PGs formed by these two isoenzymes have slightly different effects on the body. For example, some of the PGs produced by COX-1, which is normally present in the sites of inflammation and in the stomach, protect the inner lining of the stomach. Therefore, when the COX-1 enzyme is blocked, inflammation is reduced, but the protection of the lining of the stomach is lost. This can cause stomach upset as well as ulceration and bleeding from the stomach and even the intestines. However, the COX-2 enzyme is located specifically in areas of the body that commonly are involved in inflammation, but not the stomach. Therefore, when COX-2 is blocked, inflammation is reduced, but the risk of injuring the lining of the stomach is lower.

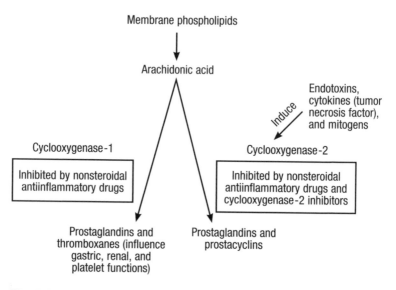

Fig. 4. Renal effects of cyclooxygenase-2 inhibitors.

CYTOKINES

Cytokines are small cell-signaling protein molecules that are secreted by the glial cells of the CNS and by numerous cells of the immune system and have a specific effect on the interactions or communications between the cells. Cytokines can be proinflammatory or antiinflammatory. Proinflammatory cytokines (interleukin-1β [IL-1β], interleukin-6, and tumor necrosis factor [TNF] are related to the pathophysiology of pain syndromes.

Cytokines have been strongly implicated in the generation of pathologic pain states at both peripheral and CNS sites. They can be broadly classified into five major groups: 1) interleukins, 2) growth factors, 3) interferons, 4) chemokines, and 5) TNF. It is known that IL-1β directly affects central sensitization by producing algesic mediators, including COX-2, inducible nitric oxide synthase, and substance P from primary afferents, which lead to persistent pain. Inhibition of proinflammatory cytokines with a cocktail of the IL-1β and TNF antagonists dramatically reduce peripheral nerve injury-induced mechanical allodynia in a dose-dependent manner. Interleukin-6 has been implicated in contributing to chronic pain after nerve injury, and TNF is primarily responsible for initiating the cascade of other cytokines in the classic immune response. Other studies also suggest the role of cytokine in hyperalgesia, opioid analgesia, and opioid tolerance (9).

Pharmacology and Physiologic Effects of Analgesics

A wide range of medications has been used to manage acute and chronic pain. This section reviews the pharmacology of the medications used for the treatment of nociceptive, inflammatory, and neuropathic pain. Some of the agents have been approved for use in humans for their analgesic actions (opioids, nonsteroidal antiinflammatory agents, and local anesthetics) and some (anticonvulsants and antidepressants) have not and are used off label.

DRUGS FOR THE TREATMENT OF NOCICEPTIVE AND ANTIINFLAMMATORY PAIN

Nonsteroidal Antiinflammatory Drugs. Most nonsteroidal antiinflammatory drugs (NSAIDs) function specifically by nonselectively but reversibly blocking the production of the enzymes COX-1 and COX-2, which inhibits the production of prostaglandins, prostacyclin, and thromboxane A_2.

The selectivity of COX-2 is expressed as a ratio of the quantity of the drug needed to inhibit the COX-1 and COX-2 enzymes by 50%. It is useful as a predictor of GI safety, but not as the determinant of overall safety for such drugs. Cyclooxygenase selectivity has little effect in predicting potential renal toxicity because both COX-1 and COX-2 are present in the kidney.

Cyclooxygenase-2 plays a complex and important role in renal pathophysiology that is not fully understood. Main adverse effects of nonselective NSAIDs include, decreased sodium excretion, decreased potassium excretion, and reduced renal perfusion. Some of these effects are also shared by selective COX-2 inhibitors, but the selectivity does not negate other adverse effects of NSAIDs, such as renal failure, and there is evidence that the risk of heart attack, thrombosis, and stroke is increased because of an increase in thromboxane levels.

Cyclooxygenase-2 inhibitors reduce the formation of prostacyclin (a potent vasodilator and platelet activation inhibitor), leaving platelet thromboxane A_2 mediated by COX-1 relatively unopposed. With a loss of the antiplatelet and vasodilatory effects of prostacyclin, a relative excess of thromboxane A_2 would favor vasoconstriction, platelet aggregation, and thrombosis.

Nonselective COX inhibitors include diclofenac, ibuprofen, indomethacin, ketorolac, and naproxen. The only NSAID of the selective COX-2 inhibitor group currently available is celecoxib. Although celecoxib carries an increased risk of cardiovascular (CV) events, the U.S. Food and Drug Administration (FDA) concluded that the benefit of celecoxib outweighs the risks in properly selected and informed patients.

Ketorolac is an NSAID with potent analgesic effects when administered intravenously or intramuscularly. It is used only for short-term pain management (up to 5 days in adults). Ketorolac, 30 mg administered intravenously, produces analgesia that is equivalent to 10 mg of morphine or 100 mg of meperidine. An important benefit of ketorolac-induced analgesia is the absence of ventilatory or CV depression. Its bioavailability is 100% after an oral dose. Maximum plasma concentration is achieved in approximately 45 minutes after oral administration and 30–45 minutes after intramuscular (IM) administration.

In general, NSAIDs are rapidly absorbed after oral administration. Their metabolism varies depending on the type of NSAID (renal or hepatic). Excretion could be renal and fecal.

Nonsteroidal antiinflammatory drugs are routinely prescribed for mild to moderate pain related to tissue disruption or inflammation. Their efficacy in treating acute pain has been well demonstrated. Also, they are effective and commonly used in the postoperative setting and for the treatment of primary and secondary dysmenorrhea. Besides their analgesic effects, NSAIDs inhibit prostacyclin production, which results in reduced menstrual blood loss in patients with menorrhagia, including those with uterine leiomyomas and adenomyosis. In the uterus, vasoconstriction is more important for hemostasis than platelet aggregation.

Most NSAIDs interfere with platelet aggregation by inhibiting the action of thromboxane A_2. With the exception of aspirin in which platelet dysfunction is permanent (or for 14 days for new platelets to be synthesized) and effects are noted for up to 7–9 days, all NSAIDs are associated with up to 2 days of reversible platelet dysfunction.

Nonsteroidal antiinflammatory drugs also have a well-established association with GI disturbances, including dyspepsia and gastroduodenal ulcer. Gastrointestinal protection can be achieved with simultaneous administration of an H_2 blocker receptor or proton pump inhibitor, such as famotidine. Furthermore, NSAIDs are known to be nephrotoxic with chronic use and should be prescribed with caution to patients with underlying kidney disease, hypertension, and heart disease and those with gastritis, gastric ulcer, or risk of GI bleeding.

Acetaminophen. Acetaminophen is an analgesic and antipyretic. Its mechanism of action has not been fully determined. Acetaminophen may act predominantly by inhibiting PG synthesis in the CNS. The peripheral action also may be caused by inhibition of PG synthesis or by inhibition of the synthesis or actions of other substances that sensitize pain receptors to mechanical or chemical stimulation. Approximately 95% of acetaminophen is metabolized in the liver by conjugation and hydroxylation and excreted by the kidney; approximately 3% is excreted unchanged.

Opioids. The term opioid refers to all exogenous substances (natural and synthetic) that bind to any of the opioid receptors and produce at least some morphine-like effects. Some of these effects may be mediated by opioid receptors on peripheral sensory nerve endings. Opioids can be classified into three categories: 1) agonists, 2) agonists–antagonists, and 3) antagonists (Table 2).

Opioid agonists produce analgesia by binding to specific brain and spinal cord receptors that are involved in the transmission and modulation of pain. These receptors are classified as mu, kappa, and delta and each has specific but overlapping functions and affinity for endogenous opioid peptides (Table 3).

Table 2. Classification of Opioids

Agonists	Agonists–Antagonists	Antagonists
Morphine	Nalbuphine — Nubain	Naloxone
Meperidine	Buprenorphine	Nalorphine
Naltrexone	Fentanyl	
Hydromorphone		
Oxymorphone		
Methadone		
Codeine		

Table 3. Opioid Receptor Subtypes and Functions

Receptor Subtype	Functions	Endogenous Opioid Affinity
mu	Supraspinal and spinal analgesia, sedation, inhibition of respiration, slowed gastrointestinal transit, and modulation of hormone and neurotransmitter release	Endorphins > enkephalins > dynorphins
delta	Supraspinal and spinal analgesia and modulation of hormone and neurotransmitter release	Enkephalins > others
kappa	Supraspinal and spinal analgesia, psychotomimetic effects, and slowed gastrointestinal transit	Dynorphins > others

Because absorption of opioids varies depending on the type of narcotic, only those most commonly used are reviewed in Table 4. Most of the metabolic processes of the opioids occur in the liver and the waste products are then excreted by the kidneys.

Although somewhat controversial in the treatment of chronic nonmalignant pain, these agents have been shown to be efficacious in a variety of pain disorders. In addition to their use for nociceptive pain, certain opioid medications also have shown effectiveness in the treatment of neuropathic pain. A 2005 review of eight studies showed significant efficacy in the improvement of neuropathic pain with long-term opioid use (median 28 days) compared with placebo (10). Oxycodone, a semisynthetic opioid analgesic agent, was studied in a small double, crossover study in 38 patients with postherpetic neuralgia (11). It was shown to produce statistically significant results in terms of reduction in overall pain and allodynia. Tramadol, a centrally acting agent with monoaminergic (serotonin and norepinephrine agonist) and opioid activity, has been studied in a double-blinded randomized controlled trial (RCT) of 131 patients with diabetic neuropathy, with statistically significant reduction in pain in the tramadol group (12). A subsequent 2007 study reported on the effects of therapy with tramadol versus placebo in more than 300 individuals with diabetic neuropathy (13) and confirmed significantly improved pain scores in patients treated with tramadol compared with placebo.

Adverse effects of opioid analgesic agents include GI upset caused by delayed gastric emptying as well as effects on the CNS and respiratory system (Box 1). Lowering of the patient's pain threshold and amenorrhea also are consequences of long-term opioid use.

Table 4. Pharmacokinetics of Opioids

Drug	Bioavailability	Peak
Morphine	Less than 40%	30 minutes
Oxycodone	60–90%	1.5 hours
Hydromorphone	Undetermined	60 minutes
Methadone	40–100%	1–7.5 hours

Box 1. Adverse Reactions to Opioids

Severe Reactions
- Respiratory depression
- Apnea
- Respiratory arrest
- Circulatory depression
- Hypotension
- Cardiac arrest
- Shock

Other Adverse Events
- Constipation
- Anorexia
- Nausea
- Vomiting
- Diarrhea
- Cramps
- Lightheadedness
- Dizziness
- Sedation
- Dysphoria
- Euphoria
- Weakness
- Headache
- Agitation
- Tremor
- Uncoordinated muscle movements
- Seizure
- Alterations of mood
- Muscle rigidity
- Transient hallucinations
- Disorientation
- Visual disturbances
- Insomnia
- Increased intracranial pressure
- Dry mouth
- Biliary tract spasm
- Taste alteration
- Ileus
- Intestinal obstruction
- Dyspepsia
- Flushing of the face
- Sweating
- Chills
- Tachycardia
- Bradycardia
- Palpitation
- Faintness
- Syncope
- Urine retention or hesitance
- Reduced libido, potency, or both
- Pruritus
- Urticaria
- Edema
- Diaphoresis
- Miosis
- Anaphylaxis
- Lowering of pain threshold
- Amenorrhea

Narcotics are contraindicated in patients with known hyper-sensitivity, patients with respiratory depression, and in patients with acute or severe bronchial asthma or hypercarbia. Relative contraindications include suspected or diagnosed paralytic ileus and renal or hepatic impairment.

Narcotics have additive effects when used in conjunction with alcohol, other opioids, or illicit drugs that cause CNS depression; respiratory depression, hypotension, and profound sedation or coma may result. Agonist–antagonist analgesics (ie, pentazocine, nalbuphine, and butorphanol) should be administered with cau-tion to a patient who has received or is receiving narcotics. In this situation, mixed agonist–antagonist analgesics may reduce the analgesic effect of narcotics, precipitate withdrawal symp-toms, or both.

Opioid dependence can develop with ongoing administration, which leads to specific withdrawal and abstinence symptoms of various levels of severity. Opioids have a potential to cause addiction and abuse in users. Further information on opioid dependence, tolerance, addiction, and abuse as well as examples of prophylactic measures are given in the section "Special Con-siderations for Medication Management."

DRUGS FOR TREATMENT OF NEUROPATHIC PAIN

Treatment of neuropathic pain is challenging. It is most likely that in patients with neuropathic pain, medications with demon-strated efficacy have not been prescribed or they have received inadequate dosages. First-line treatments for these patients are antidepressants with norepinephrine and serotonin reuptake inhibition (tricyclic antidepressants [TCAs] and serotonin–norepinephrine reuptake inhibitors [SNRIs]), calcium channel $\alpha_2\delta$-ligands (gabapentin and pregabalin), and topical lidocaine (lidocaine patch 5%) (Table 5). These medications are used off label for a wide range of neuropathic pain disorders (14).

Antidepressants. Antidepressants have been studied over the past several decades for the treatment of pain. Included within this group of drugs are TCAs, selective serotonin reuptake inhib-itors (SSRIs), and SNRIs. These agents have been determined to be efficacious for the management of chronic pain but not acute

Table 5. Drugs Used for Treatment of Neuropathic Pain

Drug	Absorption	Metabolism and Excretion	Advantages	Special Considerations
Tricyclic Antidepressants				
Amitriptyline, nortriptyline, and desipramine	Oral	Metabolism hepatic; excretion renal	Low cost, once daily dosage, and beneficial effect on depression	Anticholinergic side effects, orthostatic hypotension, cardiotoxicity, fewer side effects, and potential lower efficacy
Serotonin–Norepinephrine Reuptake inhibitor				
Duloxetine	Oral—time to peak 6–10 hours	Metabolism hepatic; excretion, 70% renal and 20% fecal	Once or twice daily dosage	Nausea
Calcium Channel α_2-δ Ligands				
Gabapentin	Bioavailability is 30–60%	Renal; entire dose is excreted unchanged		Sedation, dizziness, slow titration, and delayed onset of analgesia
Pregabalin	Bioavailability is 90%	Renal, 90%; entire dose is excreted unchanged		Shorter titration period and dose adjustment required in renal impairment
Topical Lidocaine				
Lidocaine patch, 5%	Undetectable in plasma	Hepatic, 90%, and renal,10%; the dose is excreted unchanged		Mild local irritation

pain. Only few antidepressants have been directly studied for pelvic pain. Their efficacy is thought to be related to multiple mechanisms of actions, including antidepressant activity, analgesic activity, and neurotransmitter alteration.

The effects of TCAs and presumably a new generation of antidepressant drugs have been shown to improve quality of life and symptoms of depression, particularly in people whose depressive symptoms coincided with the onset of pain symptoms (15). These agents may have a separate analgesic effect as shown in studies of patients taking TCAs that have reported an improvement in pain scores despite a lack of antidepressant response or in patients without baseline depression (15). Analgesic properties of antidepressants also may be a result of their nonspecific physiologic effects, including decreased anxiety, muscle relaxation, and restored sleep cycles.

Use of tricyclic antidepressants increases synaptic levels of dopamine, noradrenaline, and serotonin, even with short-term use. With long-term exposure at therapeutic levels, TCAs (and possibly SSRIs and SNRIs) are thought to stabilize the activity of certain neurotransmitters involved in the production of pain sensation, such as substance P and GABA. Use of TCAs is sometimes limited by their adverse effect profile, which is related to their affinity to H1 receptor, anticholinergic properties, and interaction with sodium channels. Tricyclic antidepressants with high serotonergic and noradrenergic activity, such as amitriptyline, nortriptyline, and desipramine, are particularly effective for neuropathic pain.

Tricyclic antidepressants are first-line treatment for neuropathic pain. A review identified 48 adequately conducted controlled trials of TCA use for chronic pain (16). A total of 46 of the 48 trials showed statistically significant pain relief in patients who took TCA compared with those who took placebo.

Sedation, sympathomimetic effects (tremor and insomnia), antimuscarinic effects (blurred vision, constipation, urinary hesitancy, confusion, and dry mucous membranes), CV effects (orthostatic hypotension, conduction defects, and arrhythmias), withdrawal symptoms, and weight gain have been reported as adverse effects of TCA use. Tricyclic antidepressants are competitive antagonists at muscarinic cholinergic receptors as well as strong α-adrenergic blockers, leading to both anticholinergic findings (tachycardia, dilated pupils, and dry mouth) and hypotension even at moderate doses. Ingestion of greater than 1 g of TCA is considered potentially fatal. Tricyclic antidepressants can have quinidine-like depressant effects that cause slowed conduction with wide QRS complex (duration greater than 100 milliseconds but up to 440 milliseconds). Treatment of TCA overdose includes general supportive care with possible endotracheal intubation. Cardiotoxicity (QRS complex widening) is treated with sodium bicarbonate, 50–100 mEq. Contraindications for the use of TCAs include urinary retention, closed angle glaucoma, and concurrent use of SSRIs, SNRIs, and monoamine oxidase inhibitors (MAOIs).

Serotonin–norepinephrine reuptake inhibitors, such as venlafaxine and duloxetine, provide a balanced inhibition of reuptake of serotonin and norepinephrine that is more specific than that of TCAs. A small study showed that venlafaxine may be as effective as imipramine for the treatment of pain associated with polyneuropathy (14). Serotonin–norepinephrine reuptake inhibitors have been approved by the FDA for use in the treatment of fibromyalgia, postherpetic neuropathy, and diabetic neuropathy. Their use also can improve overall quality of life in patients with chronic pain in whom depressive disorders and anxiety often coexist with chronic pain syndromes.

Adverse effects of these agents include nausea, somnolence, sweating, dizziness, sexual disturbances, hypertension, and anxiety. The use of SNRIs is contraindicated when SSRIs, TCAs, or MAOIs are used.

As the name suggests, SSRIs are believed to block the reuptake of serotonin by presynaptic neurons. In general, SSRIs tend to be less efficacious but better tolerated than TCAs for the treatment of chronic pain. They are the drug of choice for concurrent depressive and anxiety disorders. Small studies, such as a 2008 open-label trial of changes in pain severity and depressive symptoms after treatment with citalopram for 12 weeks, have suggested a trend toward pain relief with SSRIs (17). However, large controlled studies are necessary to evaluate the role of SSRIs in the treatment of chronic pelvic pain.

Gastrointestinal symptoms, decreased libido, sexual dysfunction, anxiety, insomnia, tremor, and weight gain have been reported with the use of SSRIs. Contraindications include concurrent use MAOIs, TCAs, SNRIs, or other SSRIs.

Anticonvulsants. Various anticonvulsants have been shown to be effective in the treatment of neuropathic pain. The most common anticonvulsants are gabapentin and pregabalin.

Gabapentin is a second-generation anticonvulsant. Studies have shown that the effect of gabapentin may be related to the inhibition of glutamate release from the spinal cord dorsal horn although its specific mechanism of action is unknown.

Its efficacy has been demonstrated in studies evaluating neuropathic pain with a significant reduction in average daily pain scores over an 8-week treatment period (14). Gabapentin has been shown to prevent allodynia and hyperalgesia in animal models and has been approved by the FDA for postherpetic neuralgia. Somnolence, dizziness, ataxia, headache, tremor, and weight gain are the most common adverse effects of gabapentin.

Pregabalin is a GABA analog that strongly binds to a subunit of calcium channels in CNS. Pregabalin reduces the calcium-dependent release of several neurotransmitters. However, its exact mechanism of action is unknown. The FDA-labeled indications include diabetic neuropathy, postherpetic neuralgia, and fibromyalgia. Somnolence, dizziness, and ataxia are common adverse effects. Many women report weight gain while using pregabalin. Rarely, thrombocytopenia may occur.

Local Anesthetics. Several topical analgesics have been studied for management of neuropathic pain (Table 6). One such agent, lidocaine, blocks conduction of impulses by decreasing ionic flux through the neuronal membrane. The penetration of lidocaine through intact skin will produce an analgesic effect but it is not sufficient to produce complete sensory block. Another agent, capsaicin, is a vanilloid agonist that depletes substance P from sensory nerves.

The lidocaine 5% patch and capsaicin have been proved efficacious and are approved by the FDA for the treatment of postherpetic neuralgia. These agents also have been used successfully for the management of other peripheral neuropathies, including diabetic neuropathies. Eutectic mixture of the local anesthetics lidocaine 2.5% and prilocaine 2.5% (EMLA cream) also has proved successful in small trials for treatment of peripheral neuropathy (18). Injected local anesthetics in the form of

Table 6. Dosages With Drugs Used for Neuropathic Pain

Drug	Starting Dose	Usual Effective Dose	Interval (Hours)	Adverse Effects	Drug Interaction	Comments
Amitriptyline	10–25 mg orally	50–100 mg	12–24	Cardiac dysrhythmia, somnolence, and dizziness	Tranylcypromine	
Nortriptyline	10–25 mg	50–100 mg	12–24	Cardiac dysrhythmia, somnolence, and dizziness		
Duloxetine	30 mg	60 mg	12–24	Somnolence		
Gabapentin	100–300 mg, administered once a day, with incremental dosage every 3 days	1,800–3,600 mg	8 hours	Peripheral edema, dizziness, and somnolence		Slow titration is needed, maximum dose is 3,600 mg/day, and dose adjustment is required in renal impairment.
Pregabalin	50 mg orally	200–600 mg	8 hours	Peripheral edema, dizziness, and somnolence		Shorter titration period is needed and dose adjustment is required in renal impairment.
Lidocaine patch, 5%	1–3 patches		12 hours on, 12 hours off	Skin irritation		

repeated nerve blocks have been studied in small trials and were found to have some efficacy (19).

Screening

Many women presenting with pelvic pain of greater than 6 months' duration will have a single "textbook" diagnosis and will respond to traditional gynecologic treatment. However, a substantial proportion of patients with chronic pelvic pain will have pain that is out of proportion to pathology or that does not respond appropriately to standard therapy. For example, they may have undergone surgery for an ectopic pregnancy or endometriosis and then experienced persistent pain, they may present with a series of yeast infections or urinary tract infections (UTIs) and subsequently report unrelenting pain and dyspareunia. Alternatively, they may have symptoms derived from multiple pelvic organs or experience various unexplained pain disorders. A history of depression or substance abuse also may be reported. These "red flags" should prompt the physician to consider a multidisciplinary approach, including psychologic evaluation and multimodal treatment of the chronic pain (Box 2). Screening should

 Box 2. Risk Factors for the Development of Chronic Pelvic Pain

☑ Depressive disorders

☑ Anxiety and panic disorders

☑ Stress

☑ Chronic fatigue syndrome

☑ Other comorbid pelvic pain disorders (irritable bowel syndrome, interstitial cystitis and bladder pain syndrome, and vulvodynia)

☑ Nonpelvic pain disorders (fibromyalgia, chronic headaches, myofascial pain, temporomandibular joint pain, chronic back pain, and noncardiac chest pain)

☑ Obesity

☑ Infertility

☑ Emotional, sexual, or physical trauma (past or current)

☑ Substance or alcohol abuse or use

☑ Worker's compensation or litigation issues

include focused history taking and validated questionnaires for depression, anxiety, and early trauma and substance abuse.

Counseling: Establishing a Dialogue

A physician who is treating pelvic pain should initiate an open, nonjudgmental discussion with a patient. At her initial visit with the obstetrician–gynecologist, this patient may have already seen many health care providers. She may have undergone a number of diagnostic tests and attempted a number of therapies. She may have been referred to multiple specialists, and may have even been told that the pain "is all in her head" or that nothing can be done. To ease her significant frustration, and even a sense of helplessness or hopelessness, an obstetrician–gynecologist should do the following:

- Obtain a detailed history in a systematic fashion, noting all inciting events and prior treatments.

- Describe the physiology of chronic pain, neural plasticity, pain memory, and the role of stress in lay terms. Such an approach improves the patient's ability to cope with her condition and lays the groundwork for her to accept multi-disciplinary treatment.

- Counsel the patient about lifestyle modifications to decrease her risk of persistent chronic pain, especially treatment of depression, anxiety, and substance abuse, reducing stress, avoiding of overeating and excessive weight gain, and improving poor sleep.

- Recommend psychosocial interventions in conjunction with medical and surgical treatments. Psychologic intervention is crucial especially if any of the following conditions or circumstances are present:
  —Psychopathology, especially depression or posttraumatic stress disorder
  —Substance abuse
  —Narcotic dependence
  —Significant marital discord

—Physical, emotional, or sexual abuse

—Sexual dysfunction or vaginismus

—Litigation

The most common therapies are cognitive or behavioral interventions, behavioral or relaxation therapies, and hypnosis.

Diagnosis

The evaluation of chronic pelvic pain entails obtaining a thorough history, physical examination, and appropriate use of laboratory testing, imaging, or both. The patient should be given adequate time to "tell her story." The examination must not be limited to the reproductive organs, but must include examination of the abdominal wall, lower back, pelvic floor, other pelvic viscera, and relevant nerves that supply the visceral and somatic pelvic structures and areas of pain referral.

Obtaining a Thorough History

Obtaining a detailed medical history is paramount in the evaluation of chronic pelvic pain (Box 3). It is important to address visceral, somatic, psychologic, and situational factors that may contribute to the pain. A useful chronic pelvic pain intake questionnaire can be downloaded free of charge from the International Pelvic Pain Society web site. The Beck Depression Inventory also is user friendly; a score of more than 12 suggests dysphoria and of more than 18, depression. Traumatic early life events have been identified in animal models and in humans to contribute to abnormal responses to pain as an adult and to the chronicity of pain. Physical and sexual abuse and other highly emotionally distressing events, such as the death of siblings or parents, divorce, alcoholism, or drug abuse in the family, and natural and manmade disasters (eg, wars, major industrial accidents, earthquakes, and floods) can increase vulnerability to peripheral and CNS dysregulation. Women with chronic pelvic pain manifest a significantly higher incidence of posttraumatic stress disorder than asymptomatic women in control groups. The Early Trauma Inventory Self-Report is useful for this assessment (20).

Box 3. Obtaining History for Chronic Pelvic Pain

- Chronology—When and in what context did the pain begin (postpartum, postoperative, after infection, or posttraumatic [physical, emotional, or sexual trauma])? Has the pain changed? Is it continuous or intermittent? Are any pain triggers present, such as menstrual cycle, physical activity, stress, eating, exercise, work, sleep, bowel and bladder functioning, sexual arousal, intercourse, and orgasm? What are the alleviating factors?

- Quality—What is the nature of the pain, ie, sharp, stabbing, aching, dull, and cramping? Cramping suggests muscular etiology. Burning, lancinating, or electrical pain and pain exacerbated with light touch suggest neuropathic pain.

- Severity—How is the pain rated on an analog scale (from 0 to 10, with 10 being the most severe pain imaginable)?

- Location(s)—Is the pain generalized or localized, does it exhibit radiation or dermatomal patterns, or is the pain present in the distribution of a specific nerve?

- Timing—Is the pain cyclic? Pain increased in association with the luteal phase or menstrual bleeding can suggest specific reproductive tract pathology or endometriosis or adenomyosis or provide an avenue for treatment with hormonal or menstrual suppression.

- Dyspareunia—Is dyspareunia present? The locations and circumstances of dyspareunia should be elicited. For example, entrance dyspareunia (vulvar or urethral pathology and pudendal or other neuropathy), vaginal dyspareunia (vaginal epithelial lesions, bladder or neuropathic pain, or pelvic floor trigger points or spasm), deep thrust dyspareunia (pelvic source, such as endometriosis, gastrointestinal pathology, or pelvic mass).

(continued)

Box 3. Obtaining History for Chronic Pelvic Pain
(continued)

- Genital tract symptoms—Are any symptoms present, such as abnormal vaginal bleeding, abnormal vaginal discharge, dysmenorrhea, anovulation, or pregnancy symptoms? What are the fertility status and desires of the patient? Contraception, sexually transmitted disease, past obstetric, and sexual histories should be obtained.

- Gastrointestinal symptoms—Is the pain linked with alterations in stool form or frequency, does it get worse with eating or before a bowel movement and better after a bowel movement? Is the pain accompanied by mucus or bloating? Is there dyschezia suggestive of endometriosis? Are constipation, diarrhea, flatulence, tenesmus, blood, changes in color, form, frequency, or caliber of stool present?

- Genitourinary symptoms—Is the pain accompanied by urinary frequency, nocturia, urgency, hesitancy, relief of pain with voiding, or suprapubic pain, suggestive of interstitial cystitis or bladder pain syndrome? Is dysuria, urgency, frequency, nocturia, hematuria, or incontinence present?

- Musculoskeletal symptoms—How is the pain distributed? Is it radiating? Is it associated with injury, fatigue, postural changes, exercise, and lifting (back and joint pain)? Are there many tender points?

- Neuropathic symptoms—Is burning, lancinating pain, allodynia, or numbness or weakness in distribution of a particular peripheral nerve present?

(continued)

Box 3. Obtaining History for Chronic Pelvic Pain (continued)

- Psychologic symptoms—Does the patient report depression, anxiety, trauma, or disability? Is the psychologic history significant for current and past episodes of depression or severe anxiety, hospital ization, therapies, substance and ethanol abuse and treatment, or past or current physical, sexual, or emotional abuse?

- Medication history—What medications does the patient currently use (especially those for pain and mood)? What are the doses, responses, and side effects?

- Social, educational, and work history—What is the patient's current living situation and employment status? Are disability and worker's compensation issues present? How does the pain affect the patient's social and occupational status?

- Prior evaluations and treatments for pain—What are the outcomes of prior medical and surgical treatments, including outside records, especially surgical and pathology reports, diagnostic scans, or relevant laboratory results?

- Past medical and surgical history—Are any other systemic pain conditions and autoimmune or inflammatory disorders present currently or in the past?

The patient also should be asked to fill out a daily pain rating form after her first office visit. A daily pain rating form (Box 4) provides the clinician and patient with important information for pain management. Identification of events that trigger pain, such as stress, menstruation, diet, and certain physical activities, are recorded briefly and provide insight for the patient and physician and lead to a dialogue regarding methods of pain prevention, such as dietary interventions, menstrual cycle suppression, stress reduction, pre-emptive pain medications, and physical therapy

Box 4. Pain Rating Form

Every night, note whether you had any menstrual or other vaginal bleeding on that day. Next, rate the severity of your pelvic pain on a scale from 0 (no pain) to 10 (the most severe pain imaginable). If you have two different pain locations or two different types of pelvic pain (eg, vaginal pain and right lower abdominal pain), label one as "Pain No. 1" and the other as "Pain No. 2." If you have yet another location or type of pain, you can add a column for "Pain No. 3." Make sure to note the location of each separate problem that you are tracking. Finally, document any activity, event, or feeling that you think may contribute to increasing the pain (eg, sexual intercourse, stress, housework, or exercise).

Date	Bleeding Yes/No	Pain No. 1 (0–10)	Pain No. 2 (0–10)	Pain Triggers

exercises. The improved ratings can indicate gradual improvement; or if there is no change in the pain score, the ratings can demonstrate the need to change therapy. The pain ratings can increase the patient's sense of control and decrease the feeling of helplessness. Pain is invariably increased by stress and uncertainty about diagnosis and outcome. Daily recording improves self-efficacy, demonstrates adherence, allows for diagnosis of atypical cyclic pain (luteal as opposed to just with menses), and helps the patient recognize the connection between pain and stressors. The daily pain rating form should be reviewed at follow-up visits.

Physical Examination

A complete pain-mapping physical examination should be performed with particular attention to the abdomen and back as well as vulva, vagina, pelvic floor muscles, and pelvic viscera. The pain should be reproduced with the examiner's finger and mapped to the specific location or dermatome, nerve distribution and underlying or overlying musculature assessed, and each organ palpated separately when possible. The components of a physical examination are described in Box 5. Pelvic muscles are illustrated in Figure 5 (see color plate).

Box 5. Physical Examination of a Patient With Pelvic Pain

General and Vital Signs

- A level of anxiety, general body habitus, and posture should be assessed.

- Pulse, blood pressure, weight, height and, if indicated, respiratory rate and temperature should be measured.

Abdominal

- The abdomen should be evaluated for scars and sites of hypersensitivity.

- The abdominal examination should identify myofascial trigger points and nerve entrapment. The most painful sites are localized with one finger, if possible, and marked with a pen. The sites are then evaluated with the muscles tensed. The patient should be asked to raise her head and shoulders off the table (abdominal crunch position) or raise both legs concurrently while straightened at the knees (Carnett's test). This helps to distinguish between abdominal wall pain (myofascial and neuropathic pain) and visceral pain. Abdominal wall pain is exacerbated by these maneuvers, whereas visceral pain is diminished.*

*Slocumb JC. Chronic somatic, myofascial, and neurogenic abdominal pelvic pain. Clin Obstet Gynecol 1990;33:145–53.

(continued)

Box 5. Physical Examination of a Patient With Pelvic Pain *(continued)*.

- The pubic symphysis should be palpated because tenderness may suggest pelvic girdle relaxation or rectus muscle inflammation or injury at its insertion.
- Bowel sounds and presence of masses, organomegaly, and distention are sought.
- In a standing position, the patient is examined for the presence of any hernias by palpation of the abdomen and groin with and without Valsalva maneuver.

Urogynecologic
- The vulva should be examined for lesions, rashes, atrophy, and evidence of trauma or old scars.
- A cotton-tipped swab should be used to evaluate the sites of hypersensitivity or allodynia in the vulvar vestibule.
- A pelvic examination with a speculum should be performed to inspect the cervix and vagina for irritation, hypoestrogenization, lesions, and pelvic organ prolapse and to collect samples, if indicated.
- The urethra, bladder base, vaginal side walls, pelvic floor muscles, paracervical region, and uterosacral ligaments should be palpated for any tenderness or abnormalities.
- The anterior vaginal, urethral, and trigonal areas may be palpated gently to attempt to identify pain, discharge, or thickening, which may suggest pain of urologic origin.
- Bimanual examination should be used to assess bladder tenderness and cervical motion tenderness. The uterus and adnexae also should be assessed bimanually to note abnormalities in size, shape, and mobility as well as focal tenderness.

(continued)

Box 5. Physical Examination of a Patient With Pelvic Pain

- Rectovaginal examination should be performed for uterosacral or rectovaginal tenderness, masses, or nodularity suggestive of endometriosis, malignancy, or rectal disease. Samples for occult blood testing may be collected, if indicated.

Musculoskeletal

- Evaluation of the pelvic floor should be incorporated into the urogynecologic or abdominal examination. It begins with observation of perineum and pelvic floor muscle activity during the process of squeezing and relaxation. Then pelvic floor muscle tenderness is evaluated to address a myofascial component to the pain.

Neurologic

- A focused evaluation of the patient's neurologic function should include examination of the lower abdomen, perineum, and lower extremities, if applicable for sensation of pinprick and cold. Any hyperalgesia in the distribution of a particular nerve, especially iliohypogastric, ilioinguinal, genitofemoral, pudendal, posterior femoral cutaneous, and branches of the sciatic nerve should be noted.

Laboratory Tests

Diagnostic workup includes complete blood count and, if indicated, erythrocyte sedimentation rate and pregnancy test. Clean catch midstream urinalysis and, if indicated, urine culture are recommended. The presence of squamous epithelial cells (outside the normal range as specified by the laboratory) on the urine analysis, suggests contamination with vaginal secretions and renders the specimen unsatisfactory for analysis and culture.

A Pap test, cervical studies for gonorrhea and chlamydia, wet mount testing of vaginal discharge for clue cells, trichomonads, hyphae, and estrogenization, as well as pH and amine odor test of vaginal secretions and stool guaiac test are suggested when indicated. Cystoscopy, urine cytology, and colonoscopy are indicated based on specific GU or GI symptomatology and concern for malignancy in women older than 40–50 years.

Imaging Studies

Transvaginal pelvic ultrasonography is performed to rule out structural abnormalities within the pelvis that may be missed by pelvic examination. Computed tomography (CT) with and without contrast or CT urography is helpful to rule out upper abdominal visceral pathology. The examination of the retroperitoneum and GI and GU tract evaluations are useful. Magnetic resonance imaging can be useful for the evaluation of pelvic floor and lumbar–sacral areas. Pelvic abnormalities found on ultrasound examination, especially uterine anomalies, also can be further investigated by the MRI. Magnetic resonance imaging can be used to distinguish ovarian masses from broad ligament or exophytic uterine masses. Surgical evaluation with diagnostic laparoscopy, hysteroscopy, or vulvar biopsy may be considered if pelvic examination has yielded abnormal results or therapy has failed.

Differential Diagnosis

The differential diagnosis of chronic pelvic pain is extensive and encompasses both gynecologic and nongynecologic conditions (Box 6). Gynecologic etiologies include primary dysmenorrhea, endometriosis and adenomyosis, ovarian neoplasms and functional cysts related to ovarian remnant syndrome or residual ovarian syndrome, and pelvic congestion syndrome. Pelvic adhesions (postoperative and postinfectious) often are found in women with chronic pelvic pain, but their role in pain genesis and their management is a subject of debate.

Pain syndromes that represent alterations of CNS pain modulation, such as endometriosis-related pain syndrome, myofascial pain syndrome, irritable bowel syndrome (IBS), and bladder pain syndrome are difficult to diagnose and treat. Some pain

Box 6. Differential Diagnosis of Chronic Pelvic Pain

Pelvic

- Endometriosis
- Adenomyosis
- Pelvic inflammatory disease and postinflammatory changes
- Ovarian cysts or neoplasm
- Uterine leiomyomas
- Residual ovarian syndrome
- Ovarian remnant syndrome
- Pelvic surgery or radiation damage
- Pelvic organ prolapse
- Traumatic pelvic injury
- Pelvic congestion syndrome

Vulvar and Vaginal

- Vestibulodynia
- Vulvodynia
- Vaginismus
- Atrophic epithelium, dermatoses, dermatitis, or infection
- Granuloma fissuratum of posterior fourchette
- Traumatic injury—obstetric, postoperative, and other

Musculoskeletal

- Pelvic floor muscle trigger points and dysfunction
- Myofascial pain disorder—abdominal wall, pelvic floor, or back
- Fibromyalgia

(continued)

symptoms, such as dyspareunia and vulvodynia, may be related to vulvovaginal pathology or other pelvic and sexual pain disorders.

Box 6. Differential Diagnosis of Chronic Pelvic Pain (continued)

Gastrointestinal
- Irritable bowel syndrome or functional abdominal pain syndrome
- Inflammatory bowel disease or gluten enteropathy
- Colorectal cancer

Urologic
- Urinary tract infection
- Interstitial cystitis, bladder pain syndrome, or urethritis
- Urethral diverticulum

Neurologic
- Herpes zoster
- Pudendal neuropathy
- Other neuropathy (ilioinguinal, iliohypogastric, genitofemoral, cluneal, posterior femoral cutaneous, or obturator)
- Vaginal cuff neuroma
- Multiple sclerosis or acquired immunodeficiency disorder

The somatic tissues sharing the same dermatomal distribution with the pelvic viscera are an important component of the pain process or may be the sole pain generator. Myofascial abdominal wall and pelvic floor (rectus abdominus, obliques, levator ani, and piriformis) structures often are overlooked as sources of pain. Neuropathic pain also is frequently missed and can be related to nerve entrapment by scar, tight muscles, or injury. The iliohypogastric, ilioinguinal, genitofemoral, sciatic, or pudendal nerves and their branches are vulnerable to injury and upregulation. A history of current or past emotional, sexual, or physical trauma and psychiatric disorders can affect pain presentation and treatment response.

Pharmacologic management can be specific to a particular pathology, such as dysmenorrhea, endometriosis, or nerve entrapment, or may be a part of multiplatform pain management geared toward downregulation of neural firing. Hormonal modulation also is a cornerstone in the management of chronic pelvic pain. Reproductive system pathology typically manifests as cyclic pain, with premenstrual worsening and dysmenorrhea; but nongynecologic pain often will intensify in the premenstrual and menstrual phases. Many therapeutic options currently available for cyclic pain entail suppression of the ovarian hormonal cycle or menstrual bleeding.

Pelvic Pain Disorders and Comorbidity

Reproductive, GI, and GU system pain disorders share common symptoms, and the presence of symptoms related to more than one pelvic viscera is associated with increased pain severity and disability. For example, 43% of women with IBS reported dyspareunia and 55% of women with chronic pelvic pain, IBS, and urgency or frequency of urination avoided intercourse because of pain, compared with only 22% women with chronic pelvic pain alone (4). A total of 58% of women with both chronic pelvic pain and IBS rated their pain as moderate to severe compared with 43% of women with chronic pelvic pain alone. Dysmenorrhea also was more severe if both chronic pelvic pain and IBS were present. Women with IBS are three times more likely to have had a hysterectomy or other gynecologic surgery for chronic pelvic pain and experience less improvement in pain if a laparoscopy or hysterectomy was performed for chronic pelvic pain (4).

This overlap of pain symptoms emanating from the pelvic organs and somatic tissues extends beyond the pelvis. Significant comorbidity of chronic pelvic pain and other chronic visceral and somatic functional pain and mood disorders are known to primarily affect women and include endometriosis, IBS, bladder pain syndrome or interstitial cystitis, fibromyalgia and myofascial pain, migraine, temporomandibular joint pain, chronic fatigue syndrome, generalized anxiety or panic disorders, and depression. At least 50% of patients with chronic pelvic pain or functional abdominal pain disorders have an associated psychiatric disorder and stress is most commonly reported. Emotional, sexual, and physical trauma in childhood and adulthood also are more prevalent in women with chronic pelvic pain and other "medically unexplained" pain syndromes. It has been suggested that genetic predisposition and adverse environmental pressures increase the vulnerability for and maintenance of these pain disorders (21).

Acute Pain or Chronic Pain Exacerbation

Chronic pelvic pain is defined as pelvic pain that persists in the same location for more than 6 months. The evaluation of acute pelvic pain is beyond the scope of this monograph, other than management of perioperative and end-of-life pain. However, a new acute pain process can mistakenly be interpreted by the patient and the physician as an exacerbation of a chronic pain problem. Acute pelvic pain refers to pain beginning within the week to month or so before it is reported by the patient. If the pain is not diagnosed expeditiously, it often can result in significant morbidity or mortality. Infection, rupture, or occlusion of a visceral structure, pregnancy-related complications, and carcinoma must be considered. In the setting of a recent significant chronic pain flare, especially if there is a shift in the pain location or associated symptoms, it is important to rule out a superimposed acute process, such as an ectopic pregnancy or threatened abortion, ovarian cyst with leakage or torsion, pelvic inflammatory disease (PID), UTI or ureteral calculus, appendicitis, diverticulitis, or bowel obstruction. Symptoms of fever, chills, diaphoresis, abnormal vaginal bleeding, dizziness, syncope, emesis, significant diarrhea, obstipation, dysuria, hematuria, and hematochezia or signs of elevated temperature, pulse, orthostasis, abdominal distention, abnormal bowel sounds, ascites, peritonitis, or pregnancy are suggestive of an acute process.

Management of Chronic Pelvic Pain

Pain of Urogynecologic Origin

Pain of urogynecologic origin can be categorized as cyclic and noncyclic based on the pattern of occurrence. Detailed medical history and physical examination are essential. Specific diagnoses and treatment options are outlined in this section.

CYCLIC PAIN

Pain limited to the premenstrual and menstrual phases is more likely to be of gynecologic origin than other etiologies. By definition, primary and secondary dysmenorrhea are linked with menses and the associated hormonal and inflammatory changes. However, most visceral pelvic pain syndromes, including IBS and bladder pain syndrome, often flare up premenstrually. The pain rating form includes questions on vaginal bleeding and may aid in the recognition of cyclicity of the pain. Suppression of menses or of cyclic hormonal fluctuation can be therapeutic if there is cyclic exacerbation of the pain based on history or the pain rating form. Up to 50% of menstruating women are affected by dysmenorrhea.

Primary Dysmenorrhea. Primary dysmenorrhea is defined as menstrual pain in the absence of underlying pathology. Pain typically begins with the onset of ovulatory cycles, often within a year or so of menarche. The pain is thought to be caused by increased endometrial PG production, elevated uterine tone with subsequent myometrial hypoxia, and further production of algesic substances in the uterus and CNS. The pain usually starts within hours of the onset of a menstrual period and lasts up to 72 hours. Most commonly, there is suprapubic cramping pain that radiates to the anterior thighs and lumbar–sacral region and occasionally is associated with nausea, vomiting, and diarrhea; rarely, with syncope. Physical examination yields normal results. Findings of a detailed medical history and physical and pelvic examinations typically can confirm a diagnosis of primary dysmenorrhea. Cervical studies to rule out sexually transmitted infection (STI) should be conducted. Transvaginal ultrasonography is indicated if there is suspicion of underlying pathology.

The standard initial treatment of primary dysmenorrhea is prostaglandin synthetase inhibitors. Nonsteroidal antiinflammatory drugs as well as acetaminophen have been proved effective and should be initiated at the onset of pain. Nonsteroidal antiinflammatory drugs are administered 1–3 days before onset of the menstrual period and continued around the clock for the first few days of the menstrual period. A Cochrane review found that NSAIDs were significantly more effective than placebo for pain relief (OR = 7.91) but were not found to be significantly more effective than paracetamol (acetaminophen) (22). The correct dosage

Table 7. Dosages of Nonsteroidal Antiinflammatory Drugs and Acetaminophen

Drug	Average Analgesic Dose (mg)	Interval (Hours)	Maximum Daily Dose (mg)	Comments	Compli- cations	Drug Inter- actions
Acetamino- phen	500–1,000 (orally)	4–6	3,000		Hepatotoxicity and nephrotoxicity	None
Ibuprofen	200–600 (orally)	6–8	2,400		GI discomfort, GI bleeding, nephrotoxicity, and CV– thromboembolic events	Ketorolac
Naproxen	250–500 (orally)	8–12	1,250		GI discomfort, GI bleeding, nephrotoxicity, and CV– thromboembolic events	Ketorolac
Ketorolac	30 mg initial dose and 15 mg subsequent parenteral doses (limit treatment to 5 days)	6		Use lowest effective dose or shortest duration	GI bleeding, nephrotoxicity, and CV– thromboembolic events	Other NSAIDs

Abbreviations: CV indicates cardiovascular; GI, gastrointestinal; NSAID; nonsteroidal antiinflammatory drug.

is critical because with the advent of over-the-counter availability of NSAIDs, women tend to underdose, based on product labeling (Table 7). If one NSAID fails, another should be tried because each drug affects the PG cascade differently. Disposable chemical heat patches placed on the area of referred pain are a useful supplement to NSAIDs. Acetaminophen and NSAIDs can be taken concurrently, if necessary. Occasionally, antiemetics may need to be prescribed, orally or in the form of a suppository. Limited use during menstruation of low potency oral narcotics in women with allergy or contraindications to NSAIDs or hormonal agents is reasonable.

Hormonal suppression of ovulation also is useful as primary treatment or as an adjunct to NSAIDs. The goal of therapy with hormonal contraceptives is to suppress ovulation and thin the endometrial lining. Menstrual volume is decreased and PG levels are decreased. A Cochrane review of five RCTs that assessed oral contraceptives (OCs) for the treatment of primary dysmenorrhea found OCs more effective than placebo (23). Contraceptive rings and patches and the levonorgestrel-releasing intrauterine system are presumed to be effective by the same mechanism of endometrial thinning and decreased PG production.

Any hormonal contraceptive can be administered continuously to suppress menstrual bleeding. Continuous and extended (short pill-free interval) OC regimens have a continuation rate of approximately 60% and have been shown to reduce dysmenorrhea and associated hormone withdrawal symptoms more effectively than traditional 21/7 OC regimens (24). Other effective hormonal forms of menstrual suppression include high-dose oral or depot progestins and progestin implants. Endometriosis should be ruled out in women who require more aggressive medical therapy, such as narcotic analgesia, or those with a pelvic mass.

Surgical management of primary dysmenorrhea should be considered if conservative management fails or if there is a suspicion of underlying pathology; in particular, endometriosis. Laparoscopy will rule out endometriosis but adenomyosis will not be seen at the time of laparoscopy. If laparoscopy yields negative results and there is no desire for future fertility in an older woman, hysterectomy can be considered. For nulligravid women younger than 35–40 years, hysterectomy must be preceded by extensive counseling and probably avoided in women younger than 30 years unless there are major extenuating circumstances, such as a mentally stable individual with a longstanding lack of desire for fertility or prior sterilization of the patient or her partner. Other surgical approaches to the management of dysmenorrhea include laparoscopic uterosacral nerve ablation and presacral neurectomy, but they have not been proved efficacious.

CASE NO. 1. A 17-year-old nulligravid patient presents with a 2-year history of menstrual pain that begins with day 1 of her menstrual period and lasts for 2 days. She describes the pain as severe cramping, radiating to her back, associated with occasional nausea and vomiting. The patient reports menarche at age 14 years with initially irregular menstruation that became regular after approximately 1 year. She has no other medical problems and no prior surgery. She is sexually active and uses condoms or withdrawal and reports a history of chlamydia within the past year for which she was treated with azithromycin. The patient does not have irregular bleeding, dyspareunia, diarrhea, constipation, dyschezia, or urinary symptoms. The pain is improved with ibuprofen, 200 mg every 6–8 hours as needed, but the patient feels that she is taking "too much." Physical examination reveals normal external female genitalia, vagina, and cervix. No cervical discharge is detected. Bimanual examination reveals a small, nontender, anteverted mobile uterus, no cervical motion tenderness, and no adnexal tenderness or masses.

This patient's history is strongly suggestive of primary dysmenorrhea. She reports pain symptoms strongly associated with a menstrual period and limited to the first 24–72 hours of the menstrual period. The initial onset of symptoms correlates with the onset of ovulatory cycles. Findings of her physical examination are normal. Cervical studies for chlamydia and gonorrhea are warranted, but ultrasonography is not necessary if findings of the pelvic examination are normal and there is no suspicion of secondary dysmenorrhea.

This case illustrates the importance of maximizing first-line medical management. Nonsteroidal antiinflammatory drugs can be taken in higher, more therapeutic doses; for example, ibuprofen, 600 mg every 6 hours or 800 mg every 8 hours, naproxen sodium, 550 mg every 8 hours, or mefenamic acid, 500 mg once followed by 250 mg every 6 hours. Acetaminophen also can be tried alone or with the NSAID. Medications should be administered around the clock starting with the onset of symptoms. If the adequate response is not achieved, medications can be taken 1–3 days before through the first 2–3 days of the menstrual period.

Hormonal contraception can be strongly considered in this patient, both for dysmenorrhea and birth control; however, condom use remains important for the prevention of STIs. Combined hormonal contraception—OCs, transdermal contraceptives, or vaginal ring—or depot progestins all provide a progestin-dominated thin endometrium and decreased menstrual pain. Extended regimens without a hormone-free interval are indicated if dysmenorrhea persists even when taking 21/7 contraceptive regimens. Besides pharmacologic therapy, acupuncture and transcutaneous electrical nerve stimulation (TENS) both have demonstrated efficacy for dysmenorrhea and can be recommended for patients with contraindications for or intolerance to hormonal contraception.

Secondary Dysmenorrhea. Secondary dysmenorrhea or cyclic pain secondary to underlying pathology commonly begins many years after menarche. In contrast to primary dysmenorrhea, the duration of pain is typically longer than 72 hours, often beginning 1–2 weeks before the menses and persisting until after cessation of bleeding. Etiologies include endometriosis, adenomyosis, subacute endometritis and PID, use of copper IUDs, ovarian cysts, congenital pelvic malformations, and cervical stenosis.

Endometriosis

The prevalence of endometriosis is unknown because the diagnosis requires visual confirmation. However, it is estimated to occur in approximately 10% of the general female population, in 15–20% of women with infertility, and in more than 30% of women with chronic pelvic pain (25). Endometriosis has been suggested to be the cause of pain in many adolescents with chronic pelvic pain unresponsive to medical treatment. In women with endometriosis, endometrial glands and stroma are found outside the uterine cavity, most commonly at the cul-de-sac, ovaries, and pelvic visceral and parietal peritoneum. Each menstrual cycle potentially induces further proliferation, resulting in inflammation, scarring, fibrosis, and adhesions, although not all cases of endometriosis are progressive and regression can occur spontaneously (26).

The most common symptoms include the following:

- Atypical dysmenorrhea with continuous pain or pain that starts 12 days before the menses and may involve sharp pain, pressure, or both localized to the midline but may also involve the lower abdomen, back, and rectum
- Deep thrust dyspareunia
- Subfertility
- Irregular bleeding despite ovulatory cycles
- Nongynecologic symptoms, such as cyclic dyschezia, urinary urgency, urinary frequency, bloating, and, rarely, hematochezia or hematuria.

Bimanual and rectovaginal examinations may reveal uterosacral nodularity and focal tenderness. A fixed retroverted uterus or laterally deviated cervix or uterus may be suggestive of severe disease with fibrosis. If the adnexa are involved, an ovarian cystic endometrioma may be palpated. Focal uterosacral or broad ligament area tenderness is suggestive of this condition.

Ultrasonography and MRI will not detect small implants, but endometriomas are generally distinguished by a homogenous hemorrhagic appearing cyst or cysts that do not resolve after one to two menstrual cycles. The tumor marker CA 125 is neither a specific nor a particularly sensitive marker for endometriosis. Deep endometrial biopsy of nerve endings has been suggested to have a high sensitivity and specificity for endometriosis (27), but further studies are warranted. It has been shown that the clinical diagnosis of endometriosis is accurate approximately 50% of the time. Definitive diagnosis is established surgically by laparoscopy or laparotomy. Active red flame, colorless vesicles, or petechial lesions suggest early disease whereas powder-burn, fibrotic lesions suggest more longstanding lesions. Suspicious findings should be confirmed by biopsy. Deep infiltrating lesions and peritoneal windows are most prevalent in the posterior cul-de-sac and the uterosacral ligaments and may cause pain by infiltrating the abundant nerve endings in this region (28).

The goal of medical treatment for endometriosis is to reduce the cyclic hormonal stimulation of the lesions and ultimately to decidualize or induce atrophy of the lesions. No studies have compared medical and surgical management of endometriosis. However, because of the high response, relatively low cost, and reasonable tolerability when taken with hormone therapy, an expert consensus panel has recommended a trial of NSAIDs as first-line treatment for endometriosis (29) with or without combined estrogen–progestin formulations. Both cyclic and continuous combined OCs have proved efficacious (30). Most studies have used OCs containing low-dose estrogen and androgenic progestogens; however, newer generation progestogens, such as desogestrel, appear to be equally effective.

Second-line medical therapy, including high-dose progestins or gonadotropin-releasing hormone (GnRH) analogues, often is necessary for refractory symptoms or for patients in whom estrogen use is contraindicated. However, the adverse effects of these drugs often limit their use. Progestins alone are associated with few metabolic concerns and also can be considered drugs of choice and as safe and inexpensive alternatives to surgical intervention. Contraceptives containing progestin alone or progestin plus estrogen effectively control pain symptoms in approximately three quarters of the women with endometriosis (31). The risk of recurrence of endometriosis during therapy with hormonal contraceptives is small if combined estrogen–progestin preparations or tibolone are used and unopposed estrogen is avoided.

There is little difference in the effectiveness of GnRH agonist and add-back treatment compared with other pharmacological treatments for endometriosis. Medroxyprogesterone acetate and norethindrone acetate are as effective as the GnRH analogues (32). Progestins should be administered initially in doses high enough to achieve amenorrhea. Subsequently, the doses can be decreased and tapered to control symptoms. For example, depot medroxyprogesterone acetate is best given in a dose of 150–200 mg every 2 weeks until amenorrhea occurs, then every 2–3 months as needed. Adverse effects include weight gain, acne, breakthrough bleeding, and mood changes.

Androgenic hormones, such as danazol, are thought to inhibit the luteinizing hormone surge and steroidogenesis and may have antiinflammatory effects. Also, they increase levels of free testosterone and may be associated with adverse effects, such as deepening of voice, weight gain, acne, and hirsutism. Vaginal danazol in low doses may be effective (Table 8).

Gonadotropin-releasing hormone agonists induce atrophy of the endometriosis implants through hypoestrogenism caused by downregulation of GnRH receptors. Research has shown that GnRH agonist therapy in cases of endometriosis confirmed by laparoscopy decreases the size of endometriotic lesions as well as relieves pain. Side effects are consistent with a hypoestrogenic state and include vasomotor symptoms, mood swings, vaginal dryness, decreased libido, myalgias, and bone loss. Calcium supplementation and add-back therapy with norethindrone acetate, 2–5 mg daily with or without low-dose estrogen (0.625 mg of conjugated estrogen or 1 mg of estradiol-17β), have been used successfully for preventing or reducing these adverse effects (33).

Table 8. Pharmacologic Options for Symptomatic Endometriosis

Class of Medications	Medications	Dose
Analgesics or antiinflammatory drugs	Nonsteroidal anti-inflammatory drugs	Ibuprofen, 600 mg, orally 3–4 times per day
		Naproxen sodium, 550 mg, orally twice per day
		Mefenamic acid, 500 mg initially followed by 250 mg every 6 hours
Estrogen or ovulation suppressants	Hormonal contraceptives	Cyclic or continuous regimens of oral, vaginal, or transdermal contraceptives
	High-dose progestins	Depot medroxyprogesterone acetate, 150 mg, intramuscularly every 2 weeks until amenorrhea is achieved followed by 150 mg every 3 months
		Norethindrone acetate 2–5 mg orally once per day
	Levonorgestrel-releasing intrauterine system	
	Gonadotropin-releasing hormone agonist	Leuprolide depot, 3.75 mg, intramuscularly every month or 11.5 mg, intramuscularly every 3 months
		Goserelin acetate, 3.6 mg subcutaneous implant every month
	Danazol	100 mg, orally twice per day should be titrated over 3–6 months to a maximum of 200 mg four times per day or 400 mg, orally twice per day; alternatively, 200-mg vaginal suppositories (compounded) nightly
	Aromatase inhibitor	Letrozole, 2.5 mg, orally once per day (with cycle suppression; eg, norethindrone, 5–10 mg, once per day or oral contraceptives)

The side effect profile limits the use of GnRH to 8–12 months, but in some circumstances with the use of add-back hormones, bisphosphonate, or both, GnRH therapy can be used for more than 1 year. Recurrence of symptoms after discontinuation of

GnRH agonist treatment ranges from 36% to 70% at 5 years after completion of treatment.

A randomized controlled trial of the levonorgestrel-releasing intrauterine system and depot GnRH for the treatment of chronic pain related to endometriosis found that both were effective treatments and one was not significantly better than the other (34).

An important pathway that appears to be involved in the genesis of endometriotic implants is P450–prostaglandin E_2 aromatase. Aromatase plays an important role in estrogen biosynthesis by catalyzing the conversion of androstenedione and testosterone to estrone and estradiol. Although aromatase activity is not detectable in normal endometrium, it is expressed in eutopic endometrium and endometriotic lesions. In addition, estrogen is known to upregulate prostaglandin E_2, which in turn further increases aromatase activity in endometriotic cells, leading to a cycle of repeated proliferation and inflammation. As a result of these findings, aromatase inhibitors are now being used as adjunctive therapy to first-line medical therapy in refractory cases. A 2008 review of eight studies (a total of 137 women) evaluated outcomes of aromatase inhibitors for management of endometriosis. Among case series or reports (including seven studies with a total of 40 women), aromatase inhibitors combined with progestins or OCs or GnRH analogues reduced mean pain scores and lesion size and improved quality of life. In the only reviewed RCT (including 97 women), use of an aromatase inhibitor (anastrozole) in combination with a GnRH agonist significantly improved pain ($P<.0001$) compared with use of a GnRH agonist alone at the time of the 6-month follow-up and there was no significant reduction in spine or hip bone density (35). A 2009 open-label nonrandomized trial evaluated 82 women with rectovaginal endometriosis who received either letrozole plus norethindrone or norethindrone alone. After 6 months of therapy, intensity of pain and deep dyspareunia were significantly lower in the letrozole group, but letrozole also produced more adverse effects than norethindrone alone. Furthermore, at 6 months after completion of therapy, there was no difference in pain scores between the two groups (36).

Progesterone antagonists, such as mifepristone (RU486), have been shown to block progesterone receptors in endometriotic tissue, thus impairing functional integrity and shedding. Early clinical work showed some benefit of mifepristone in improving endometriosis-associated pain, at a dose of 100 mg daily for 3 months. Mifepristone reduced pelvic pain in a small pilot study, but erratic vaginal bleeding was a problem. Further work is required to confirm these data and to minimize adverse effects (37).

Selective estrogen receptor modulators (SERMs), such as raloxifene, have been shown to suppress proliferation of endometriotic tissue and have been used safely in menopausal women for other indications. New SERMs for the treatment of endometriosis have shown some promise in animal studies with significant regression of endometriotic implants. However, human studies are necessary to confirm efficacy and safety (38).

Statins are cholesterol-lowering agents that inhibit the activity of human menopausal gonadotropin–coenzyme A reductase. In vitro data suggest that statins can inhibit the growth of human endometrial cells by inhibition of this pathway (39). These early data require confirmation from further basic and clinical studies. Selective progesterone receptor modulators and angiogenesis inhibitors also are under investigation as potential treatment options. Other novel approaches to management that are currently under investigation include use of antiangiogenic drugs to target vascular endothelial growth factor and immunomodulators to target tumor necrosis factor α (38).

Laparoscopy and laparotomy are appropriate and in some settings should be used as first-line interventions for the management of pain related to endometriosis. Failure to respond to therapy with hormonal contraceptives can suggest the pain is not due to endometriosis, although deeply infiltrating disease, particularly in the cul-de-sac, is less likely to respond to medical therapy or superficial ablation. Considerable laparoscopic skill is required to manage this form of disease, and in many European countries with nationalized health care, these cases are referred to regional specialists and are not managed by general obstetrician–gynecologists.

At the time of laparoscopy, endometriotic lesions should be ablated or resected. Endometriomas should be removed with their capsule. Resection of endometriomas by ovarian cystectomy improves pain relief as well as pregnancy rates in women with a history of chronic pelvic pain and endometriosis when compared with fenestration, drainage, and coagulation. The benefits of laparoscopy over laparotomy are well known in terms of decreased postoperative morbidity and recovery time. In an RCT of laser ablation for the treatment of minimal to moderate endometriosis, more than 90% of women noted improvement at 1-year follow-up and 87% of women with stage III to stage IV endometriosis were satisfied with results at 1-year follow-up. Recurrence rate of pain after 24 months is close to 50% (40).

In women who no longer desire fertility preservation, hysterectomy with bilateral salpingo-oophorectomy and removal of endometriosis lesions are recommended. If reasonable, one ovary should be preserved in women younger than 40 years, especially in those with objections or contraindications to therapy with hormonal contraceptives. Hysterectomy without bilateral salpingo-oophorectomy is associated with a higher rate of disease recurrence and a 30% reoperation rate than hysterectomy with bilateral salpingo-oophorectomy.

Limited data exist regarding the short- and long-term outcomes for repeated conservative surgical procedures, including the study on efficacy of pelvic denervating procedures (40). The authors conclude that although reoperation often is considered the best option, the long-term outcome appears suboptimal with a cumulative probability of pain recurrence between 20% and 40% and of a further surgical procedure of at least 20%. Hysterectomy for pain associated with endometriosis resulted in reasonable relief although approximately 15% of patients had persistent symptoms and pain was exacerbated in up to 5% of patients. Hysterectomy with bilateral salpingo-oophorectomy reduced the need for reoperation because of pelvic pain sixfold. Postoperative medical treatment administered for a few months is not particularly effective, and the information on prolonged combined contraceptive or progestin-alone therapy is limited. Reoperation in a symptomatic patient after previous conservative surgery should take into account the psychologic state of the patient and desire for imminent conception and future fertility and whether the pain adequately responded to prior surgical therapy (at least 1 year, but preferably 3–5 years of pain relief). If the patient has declined medical therapy or if the medical therapy failed, if she has no other untreated, comorbid visceral or somatic pain conditions or psychologic morbidity, and if she responded appropriately to prior surgery, reoperation can be recommended.

> **CASE NO. 2.** A 26-year old nulligravid woman presents with a 3-year history of pelvic pain. She describes the pain as cramps in the suprapubic area and sharp right lower quadrant, with a score of 6 out of 10 in severity, and fairly constant. She states she has more painful days than pain-free days each month and the pain worsens premenstrually and during the menstrual period. She has some deep dyspareunia and uses ibuprofen as prescribed. The patient states she has missed several days of work over the past 2 months because of severe pain. She has some depression and has noted new onset of headaches and low back pain. On examination, the abdomen is nontender without masses. The area of pain in the right lower quadrant is less tender with a straight leg raise maneuver. Pelvic floor muscles are tight and tender. Uterus is retroverted and nontender; its size and shape are normal. The adnexa are without masses or tenderness. Rectovaginal examination reveals some tenderness of uterosacral ligaments. Pelvic ultrasonography and STI work-up yield negative results. A daily pain calendar is helpful to confirm the cyclic nature of her pain.

The primary diagnosis is endometriosis, but myofascial pain is in the differential and depression is of concern as a modulating factor. Initially, maximized first-line treatment with appropriate regimens of at least two different NSAIDs should be ensured. A trial of hormonal contraception, cyclic or extended regimen, is considered first-line therapy because the patient does not wish to conceive in the near future. Pelvic floor muscle physical therapy should be recommended if available. Referrals for psychologic and psychiatric evaluation of depression and cognitive behavioral therapy, psychotherapy, or pharmacologic therapy are indicated, as is a referral to a primary health care provider for headaches. If there has been no substantial improvement after 3–6 months of first-line therapy, second-line agents, such as a GnRH analogue with progestin (for example, norethindrone acetate, 5 mg daily) for vasomotor symptoms or danazol are recommended. Alternatively, diagnostic laparoscopy should be performed at this time. If endometriosis is found during laparoscopy, the patient may still need to continue physical therapy and treatment of depression, especially if pain persists after adequate surgical excision of endometriosis. Cognitive behavioral pain management and acupuncture also can be initiated and menstrual suppression with hormonal contraceptives or progestins should be continued.

Rectovaginal endometriosis often is deeply infiltrating, highly innervated, typically associated with considerable pelvic pain, and can be a surgical challenge for laparoscopic resection. Hormonal therapy is a viable option. A study reviewing use of hormone therapy included 68 patients in five observational studies, 59 patients in a cohort study, and 90 patients in an RCT (41). The review compared the effectiveness of aromatase inhibitor, vaginal danazol, GnRH agonist, intrauterine progestin, and two estrogen–progestin combinations, transvaginally or transdermally, and an oral progestin. With the exception of an aromatase inhibitor used alone, the pain relief afforded by the medical therapies was high during the course of treatment, which ranged from 6 months to 12 months, with 60–90% of women reporting substantial reduction in pain or complete relief from pain symptoms.

Endometriosis-related pain syndrome is a new and evolving concept that can be considered when pain does not respond adequately to appropriate medical and surgical therapy, especially in the setting of minimal or mild disease. In this situation, neural plasticity results from central sensitization, which is hypothesized to be related to the peripheral inflammatory insult, and the disease is no longer the endometriosis, but the chronic pain itself. Because endometriosis-related pain syndrome often coexists with bladder pain syndrome and interstitial cystitis, IBS, myofascial pain, fibromyalgia, and vulvodynia, these disorders will need to be investigated and managed concurrently. Pelvic pain is more likely to be caused by endometriosis, if the following criteria are met (42):

1. Surgical confirmation (affected glands and stroma on histology)
2. Cyclic pain
3. Appropriate response to medical or surgical management

Adenomyosis

Adenomyosis refers to the presence of ectopic endometrial glands and stroma within the myometrium. Histologic evaluation of a hysterectomy specimen is required for definitive diagnosis, and the diagnosis often is based on clinical suspicion.

Hysterectomy is the only definitive treatment of adenomyosis. Conservative medical management improves symptoms, and should be employed before surgical therapy. The mainstay of medical management involves hormonal suppression with hormonal contraceptives, high-dose progestins, intrauterine progestin-secreting devices, GnRH agonists, or hormonal contraceptives with aromatase inhibitors. Uterine artery embolization has showed promise for women not desiring conception.

Ovarian Remnant Syndrome

Ovarian remnant syndrome is a rare complication of salpingo-oophorectomy, in which ovarian cortical tissue is left in situ, often becoming retroperitoneal. The remaining ovarian tissue may become cystic and lead to pain. Typically, it is associated with difficult surgery with intraoperative findings of extensive intraperitoneal inflammation from tubo–ovarian abscesses or endometriosis. Ovarian remnant syndrome is characterized by cyclic pelvic pain that may be chronic. Onset of pain usually is within the first 5 years of surgery. Associated flank pain, and at times, GU, GI, or both types of symptoms may be present. Pelvic examination may reveal a tender mass in the lateral region of the pelvis. Diagnosis is based on history and findings of the physical examination, ultrasonography, and hormonal evaluation. If the patient has had bilateral salpingo-oophorectomy and is not using hormone therapy, estradiol and follicle-stimulating hormone levels usually are in premenopausal range. Clomiphene citrate, 50 mg for 5 days, has been used to stimulate the remnant ovarian tissue for enhanced visualization. The ultrasound examination should be performed 7 days after the conclusion of the clomiphene citrate administration.

Surgical management with removal of all suspicious tissue is the treatment of choice for definitive resection of the residual ovarian tissue. Laparoscopic management is controversial because ovarian remnant syndrome usually is associated with extensive intra-abdominal adhesions that increase the risk of additional complications, such as bowel, bladder, or ureteral injury. The recurrence rate may be as high as 15% after surgical management. This syndrome also can be managed conservatively with hormonal suppression. Suppression with GnRH agonists has been shown to be superior with respect to improvement of pain compared with other methods, such as OCs, progestins, or danazol.

Residual Ovary Syndrome

Residual ovary syndrome is the name given to a chronic pain condition related to recurrent large functional ovarian cysts with ovaries encased in adhesions in women who have undergone hysterectomy. In these cases, one or both ovaries may be adherent to the pelvic sidewall or vaginal cuff and cause pain that usually is cyclic in nature and associated with cyst formation. Cysts measure 4–8 cm and generally resolve and reform. Dyspareunia is common. Physical examination may reveal a pelvic mass or tenderness laterally at the pelvic sidewall or in the area of the vaginal cuff. Ultrasonography may reveal a pelvic mass. The mass usually resolves and recurs within a few months.

Ovarian suppression is the mainstay of management of residual ovarian syndrome. Combined hormonal contraceptives and high-dose progestins have been used successfully in the treatment of residual ovary syndrome. Salpingo-oophorectomy may be necessary in refractory cases in patients who do not wish to use hormonal contraceptives, or in patients with contraindications.

NONCYCLIC GYNECOLOGIC PAIN

Ovarian Cysts and Adnexal Masses. Ovarian cystic and solid neoplasms, ie, benign and malignant and functional cysts (follicles and corpus luteal cysts), usually are asymptomatic unless there is rapid expansion of the capsule, leakage of an irritating substance (blood and dermoid or endometrioma contents), torsion with occlusion of blood supply, or infection. In these cases, acute and rapidly escalating pain with associated nausea, emesis, syncope, diaphoresis or fever, and peritoneal signs may ensue.

Adnexal masses are associated with acute pain from torsion or rupture. However, they may cause chronic pain symptoms if they are large enough to encroach on adjacent pelvic structures, such as the bladder and bowel or are compressed during sexual intercourse. Physical examination and pelvic ultrasonography will reveal a pelvic mass.

The management of chronic pain with an adnexal mass is beyond the scope of this monograph. However, in reproductive-aged women, unilateral simple or hemorrhagic masses smaller than 6–8 cm without acute potentially morbid symptoms often emerge as functional cysts and should be managed expectantly, not surgically, for 6–8 weeks. On repeat ultrasonography, if the cyst is persistent, surgery is indicated.

Uterine Leiomyomas. Uterine leiomyomas are the most common pelvic mass, occurring in 20% of women; 30% of these women will experience mild pain and discomfort from direct pressure on the bladder, bowel, or supporting ligaments. Leiomyomas cause acute severe pain if degeneration occurs from a reduced blood supply and infarction, usually in the setting or from pregnancy or torsion.

Pelvic Congestion Syndrome. Pelvic congestion syndrome refers to the congestion or dilation of uterine venous plexuses, ovarian venous plexuses, or both. Dull pelvic aching with acute, severe exacerbations, often worsened with prolonged standing and sexual activity, have been described.

All other etiologies of chronic pelvic pain should be ruled out before the diagnosis can be established. Management strategies have shown mixed results. Gonadotropin-releasing hormone agonists, high-dose progestins, cognitive behavioral therapy, hysterectomy with oophorectomy, and possibly ovarian vein embolization have all shown some efficacy. A randomized controlled trial that compared treatment with a GnRH agonist and treatment with oral medroxyprogesterone demonstrated increased efficacy of GnRH as reported 1 year after completion of treatment (43). A more recent RCT showed no difference between GnRH agonist with norethindrone add-back therapy compared with oral contraceptives in the treatment of endometriosis-related pelvic pain (44).

Transcatheter embolization of pelvic veins has shown some promise based on the results of a few small uncontrolled studies, but larger RCTs are necessary to confirm its benefit. In a

2006 study, 131 women underwent transfemoral venography for strong clinical suspicion of pelvic congestion (45). The diagnosis was confirmed in 127 of these women. Internal iliac embolotherapy was performed in 108 women. Ninety-seven patients completed long-term clinical follow-up (mean 45 months plus or minus 18 months). The mean pelvic pain level had improved significantly from a score of 7.6 plus or minus 1.8 before embolotherapy to a score of 2.9 plus or minus 2.8 after embolotherapy (P<.0001). Significant improvement in each category of specific symptoms also was noted (P<.0001). Overall, 83% of the patients exhibited clinical improvement at long-term follow-up, 13% had no significant change, and 4% exhibited a worsened condition. No significant change was noted in hormone levels after embolotherapy. Hysterectomy with bilateral salpingo-oophorectomy is sometimes considered for refractory cases, but at least one prospective study noted residual pain in one third of those women who did not experience adequate relief from the use of hormonal therapy and subsequently underwent surgical management (46).

Pelvic Inflammatory Disease. Although PID typically presents as an acute process, chronic pain can develop in cases of subacute polymicrobial infection triggered by chlamydia. Chronic pain also may be related to resultant past salpingo-oophoritis with hydrosalpinges or by an inflammatory insult, leading to chronic upregulation of neural processing. If tissue distortion is playing a role in the pain, adhesiolysis and salpingectomy for the hydrosalpinx may be helpful and improve the outcome of in vitro fertilization. However, RCTs of adhesiolysis generally demonstrate a less than optimal outcome for pain relief.

Patients may have mild to moderate generalized lower abdominal pain, sometimes attributed to IBS. Chlamydia or gonorrhea polymerase chain reaction (PCR) results may be positive. The diagnosis of acute PID is established by clinical criteria. Two of the following major criteria must be present:

1. Lower abdominal pain and tenderness with or without rebound
2. Cervical motion tenderness
3. Adnexal tenderness

Furthermore, one of the six minor criteria must accompany the major criteria:

1. Temperature greater than 38°C
2. Leukocytosis (white blood cell count greater than 10,500)
3. Culdocentesis fluid containing white blood cells and bacteria on gram stain analysis
4. Presence of an inflammatory mass
5. Elevated erythrocyte sedimentation rate
6. Identification of gonorrhea or chlamydia from an endocervical specimen

Patients with recurrent pelvic pain in whom persistent or repeated episodes of subacute or chronic PID has been diagnosed should undergo laparoscopy because the diagnosis is likely to be incorrect, and often endometriosis is found.

Adhesions. The association between adhesions and chronic pelvic pain remains controversial. The mechanism by which adhesions lead to chronic pelvic pain is thought to be related to restriction of pelvic organs or decreased bowel motility and subsequent distention. However, study outcomes vary widely. The incidence of adhesions in patients undergoing laparoscopy for chronic pelvic pain varies from 16% to 51%. A retrospective study of 100 consecutive trials of laparoscopy found adhesions in 26% of patients with chronic pelvic pain and in 39% of asymptomatic patients with infertility, without significant differences in location or density of adhesions between the two groups. Given several studies with similar results, one cannot conclude a causal relationship between adhesions and chronic pelvic pain (47).

Patients with pain attributed to adhesions may report constant, noncyclic pelvic pain and dyspareunia. Bowel obstruction symptoms and signs may be present in severe cases. Uterine immobility may be present on examination. Laparoscopy or laparotomy is the mainstay of diagnosis. A technique called pain mapping that involves microlaparoscopy with local anesthesia and conscious sedation has not proved useful for pain management. In an observational study of 50 women undergoing pain mapping, manipulation of adhesions was observed to contribute to pain (48). However, adhesiolysis of these areas did not improve long-term pain outcomes.

Because the true relationship of adhesions to pelvic pain is
unclear, studies of adhesiolysis remain equally controversial.
Several retrospective, uncontrolled studies suggest improvement
of pain symptoms in 50–90% of patients. However, a 2003 RCT
found that adhesiolysis did not result in significant benefit compared with expectant management in women with mild to moderate adhesive disease (49). This study evaluated 100 patients with
chronic pelvic pain who were randomly assigned to either laparoscopic adhesiolysis or diagnostic laparoscopy alone. Patients were
not informed of their group status for 1 year after laparoscopy.
Both groups reported substantial pain relief and a significantly
improved quality of life, and there was no difference between
the groups as demonstrated by the mean change from baseline
of pain visual analog score at 12 months (difference 3 points;
$P=.53$; 95% CI, –7 to 13). A few small uncontrolled studies have
suggested that right-sided paracolic adhesiolysis may confer
further benefit in pain reduction. However, these adhesions occur
in most patients without pain and are generally believed to be
physiologic. One article that critically evaluated the methodology
and conclusions of several small trials asserted that all studies available at this time have been insufficiently powered (50).
Additional large RCTs are needed and one is currently underway
in the United Kingdom.

Pelvic Organ Prolapse*.* Pelvic organ prolapse results from herniation of a pelvic organ (uterus, vaginal apex, bladder, and
rectum) through the vaginal walls and into the vaginal compart-
ment. Associated factors include multiparity, large infant size,
operative vaginal delivery, obesity, advanced age, estrogen
deficiency, neurogenic dysfunction, connective tissue disorders,
prior pelvic surgery, and chronically increased intra-abdominal
pressure, such as associated with ascites, chronic cough, chronic
constipation, or occupations requiring chronic repetitive lifting or
straining.

Women with prolapse report a sensation of pressure, fullness,
or heaviness. They may note a vaginal bulge that protrudes
beyond the hymenal opening that causes discomfort with activity.
The prolapse may be relieved by lying down. Severe incapacitat-
ing pain is not, as a rule, due to prolapse. A large anterior vaginal
prolapse (cystocele) with vaginal vault eversion can lead to urinary

retention. Posterior vaginal prolapse (rectocele) can cause defeca-
tory dysfunctions, such as constipation and bowel evacuation
difficulties. Severe constipation can increase pain related to
dysmenorrhea or GI pathology. Pelvic organ prolapse can be
associated with dyspareunia, but studies found that dyspareunia
does not vary based on the grade of prolapse. Protrusion of the
vaginal epithelium can cause irritation and discomfort.

Surgery is the mainstay of treatment, although studies demonstrate recurrence or reoperation rates of up to 30% (51). The
traditional combination of Burch colposuspension for the treatment of urinary incontinence with posterior colporrhaphy has
an increased incidence of postoperative dyspareunia. Levator ani
muscle plication also can result in narrowing of the mid-vagina
region and result in a high percentage of postoperative dyspareunia. However, most posterior vaginal repair surgery helps relieve
symptoms of painful intercourse and constipation. Mesh placement to augment vaginal repairs can have painful complications.
Postoperative pain and dyspareunia can occur if lateral attachments are incorrectly placed and encroach on the pudendal nerve
or if there is mesh contraction or exposure through the vaginal
epithelium or erosion into surrounding viscera.

Vault suspension overall improves dyspareunia. Hysterectomy
for prolapse overall improves dyspareunia and pelvic discomfort, regardless of the approach. Care must be taken to ensure
appropriate vault support to preserve vaginal length. In some
cases, pain during intercourse can be exacerbated by surgery.
Pelvic floor muscle exercises, physical therapy, and behavioral
modification should all be considered to treat women with
lesser degrees of prolapse. Pessaries can be used in women with
prolapse who are not surgical candidates or who would prefer
nonsurgical approaches.

Vaginal Cuff Neuroma. After hysterectomy, patients can develop
dyspareunia due to vaginal apex pain and cuff neuroma. Vaginal
cuff neuromas are extremely rare, although the exact incidence
is unknown. Excision of the vaginal apex can provide pain relief
for these patients, especially when used in conjunction with
local anesthetic injections. Local anesthetic infiltration alone can
be diagnostic and also therapeutic. Although vaginal apex resection is effective for dyspareunia caused by neuroma, this pain

relief may be temporary, and continued medical therapy with anticonvulsants or antidepressants may be needed.

UROLOGIC CAUSES OF CHRONIC PELVIC PAIN

The urinary and reproductive systems develop in close proximity embryologically; they are derived from the urogenital sinus, which in turn gives rise to the bladder trigone and vestibule. These anatomic relationships as well as the complex interaction between the thoracolumbar and sacral autonomic innervations of both systems result in frequent overlap between pelvic and perineal pain with bladder pain and irritative voiding symptoms, such as recurrent infectious cystitis, urethral syndrome, interstitial cystitis, and bladder pain syndrome.

Recurrent Infectious Cystitis. Symptoms include suprapubic pain, dysuria, frequency and urgency, hesitancy, and sometimes hematuria. Laboratory testing, including complete urinalysis and gonorrhea and chlamydia PCR, is recommended. Antibiotic treatment is indicated based on sensitivities. Test of cure culture 7 days later should be performed to rule out persistent infection. Perimenopausal and postmenopausal women may benefit from vaginal estrogenization, altering the vaginal pH and modifying vaginal flora. Women with a history of postcoital infections benefit from postcoital voiding and prophylactic antibiotics.

Urethral Syndrome. Irritative lower urinary tract symptoms, such as dysuria, suprapubic discomfort, urinary frequency, and dyspareunia, have been reported with this condition. Slow and painful discharge of urine may be present. A thorough physical examination is performed to evaluate for possible structural causes of pain. The urethra also should be evaluated for gonorrhea and chlamydia. Urethral pain also can be a manifestation of vulvodynia or bladder pain syndrome and interstitial cystitis. Antibiotics for infection and pelvic floor muscle biofeedback aimed at modifying voiding habits are the recommended treatments for urethral syndrome.

Interstitial Cystitis and Bladder Pain Syndrome. Interstitial cystitis and bladder pain syndrome are well known causes of pelvic pain and dyspareunia, but the widespread prevalence is underappreciated. In 2008, the European Society for the Study of Interstitial Cystitis suggested the term bladder pain syndrome to replace the term interstitial cystitis because cystoscopy, a diagnostic element of the National Institute of Diabetes and Digestive and Kidney Diseases diagnostic criterion for interstitial cystitis, was encumbered by many false-positive and false-negative results. *Bladder pain syndrome* refers to chronic pelvic pain, pressure, or discomfort thought to be related to the bladder pain with at least one other urinary symptom, such as urinary frequency or persistent urge to void, with the exclusion of other disorders, such as infection, radiation, or neoplasia (52). Often these two conditions are referred to collectively as interstitial cystitis/bladder pain syndrome (IC/BPS) to include all cases of urinary pain that cannot be attributed to other causes, such as infection or urinary stones. The prevalence of IC/BPS varies widely from 20–500 patients per 100,000 population, but may be even higher based on more recent studies that evaluated an expanded definition of the condition (53). It is an easy diagnosis to overlook because many women present with atypical symptoms, eg, vulvodynia, dyspareunia, vaginal pain, and pelvic pain, and also because urinary frequency in women often is considered normal. Additionally, a high prevalence of coexisting endometriosis accompanies this disorder. Once the endometriosis is found and treated, the gynecologist may assume the problem was solved, only to find the patient still has pain and urinary symptoms. Sometimes another hormonal medication or surgery is recommended without recognizing the urologic diagnosis. Urologists also can overlook the diagnosis. They may perform an office cystoscopy and if the results are normal they refer the patient to a gynecologist. However, even normal results of cystoscopy under anesthesia with hydrodistention do not rule out bladder pain syndrome.

The etiology remains unclear, but several theories exist:

1. Defective epithelial barrier, specifically a glycosaminoglycan layer that allows irritative substances in the urine to permeate the urothelium to the subepithelial nerve endings. Most women who experience interstitial cystitis have a positive potassium diffusion test result (the test will be discussed later) and are sensitive to certain foods and beverages.

2. Abnormal mast cell activity and increased numbers of substance P expressing nerve fibers and increased nerve growth factor, all of which have been found in bladder biopsies of individuals affected by interstitial cystitis

3. Systemic autoimmune mechanism with bladder manifestations because there is a high incidence of systemic lupus erythematosus, allergies, inflammatory bowel disease, IBS, and fibromyalgia

4. Central sensitization has been suggested on the basis of altered sympathetic and hypothalamic adrenal axis in humans and in the animal models. Furthermore, there is "phantom pain," ie, even after removal of the bladder, the pain persists. Additionally, no identifiable organism or toxin has ever been found, and the findings of the glycosaminoglycan examination are inconclusive.

The diagnosis is one of exclusion. Exclusion criteria include the following factors:

- Age younger than 18 years
- Duration less than 9 months
- Absence of nocturia
- Frequency less than eight times per day
- Genitourinary infection (including bacterial cystitis, vaginitis, and herpes)
- Radiation therapy and chemotherapy
- Bladder calculi
- Genitourinary cancer
- Lack of urgency with bladder filled by greater than 350 cm^3 of urine
- Involuntary bladder contractions
- Relief with antibiotics, antispasmodics, or anticholinergics

National Institutes of Health Consensus Criteria state that at least two of the following criteria are needed for the diagnosis of interstitial cystitis:

- Pain on bladder filling relieved by emptying
- Pain in suprapubic, pelvic, urethral, vaginal, or perineal region

- Glomerulations on endoscopy or decreased compliance on cystometrogram

Further evaluation includes cystoscopy with hydrodistention and biopsy. Petechial bladder mucosal hemorrhages (glomerulations) are characteristic.

Although not currently used as diagnostic criteria, urodynamic studies may provide useful information in distinguishing IC/BPS from other urologic conditions associated with urgency and frequency. Retrospective study of urodynamic testing in women with IC/BPS compared with women with overactive bladder syndrome found significant differences in test results between the two groups, specifically in terms of reduced volume of maximum cystometric capacity and reduced volumes at each interval in women with IC/BPS (54). Reduced bladder capacity (less than 250 cm^3) is less common but may suggest more severe disease.

Patients without the cystoscopic findings of glomerulations are theorized to have a different form of interstitial cystitis, called bladder pain syndrome, whereby the pain is not caused by bladder inflammation but by an abnormal, augmented central and peripheral pain response to bladder filling and irritants. Pelvic floor myalgia and dysfunction and vulvodynia are common. Pain can be present even after surgical removal of the bladder.

Urine analysis should be performed to rule out infection. In women older than 50 years or in those with hematoma, urinary cytology and cystoscopy are indicated to rule out malignancy.

The potassium chloride (KCl) instillation test has been used with some success but has not been generally accepted as a standard test (55). The test yields positive results in 70–90% of patients with interstitial cystitis, but false positive-results are a problem. It is performed as follows: the bladder is filled with 40 mL of sterile water by a 10 Fr pediatric feeding tube, the water is held for 5 minutes, and the pain and urgency are rated with a score ranging from 0 to 5 (5 being the most severe). The water is drained and 40 mL of KCl (20 mEq KCl in 50 mL water) is instilled and held for up to 5 minutes. Again, the pain is rated and the solution is drained. Urgency or pain with a score of 2 or higher indicates a positive KCl test result. The test itself is painful and often requires instillation of a local anesthetic "cocktail" containing 100 mL of normal saline solution with 20,000 units of heparin, 16 mL of 2% lidocaine, and 3 mL of 8.4% sodium bicarbonate. Some clinicians have substituted the KCl test with a trial of this local anesthetic bladder instillation. If the anesthetic immediately relieves the pelvic pain, the bladder is believed to be involved in the etiology of pain.

Although there is no definitive cure for IC/BPS, prolonged remissions can be obtained. Table 9 summarizes the treatment modalities available for IC/BPS. First-line treatments include behavioral modification, physical therapy, and pharmacologic approaches (56). Urinary alkalinization can be helpful (57). Local treatment of dysuria and dyspareunia associated with interstitial cystitis has been proved to be effective. Tricyclic antidepressants also have been used with good efficacy. Oral pentosan polysulfate sodium has shown promise and is the only oral therapy for interstitial cystitis approved by the FDA, but it must be used for at least 6 months. Pentosan polysulfate sodium is a heparin-like moiety that resembles the glycosaminoglycan layer, but it should not be used with NSAIDs because of the bleeding risk.

Intravesical therapy can be used as a first- or second-line modality. With an intravesical mixture of lidocaine, bicarbonate, and heparin instilled three times a week for 3 weeks, 57% of patients reported resolution of pain (58). Dimethyl sulfoxide (DMSO) is the only FDA-approved intravesical treatment for interstitial cystitis. Intravesical 50% DMSO has shown significant symptomatic improvement compared with placebo in two RCTs (59, 60). A typical treatment regimen is a weekly instillation of 50 mL of 50% DMSO for 6 weeks followed by maintenance therapy every 2–4 weeks with the goal of spacing maintenance to every 2–3 months. Intravesical solutions that contain dissolved pentosan polysulfate sodium have shown some promise but are not FDA approved and are currently under investigation (61).

Cyclosporine also has shown promise in cases of severe interstitial cystitis; however, the side effect profile limits its use to patients with severe, refractory disease who can be closely monitored. A small study showed that lumbar epidural local anesthetic nerve blocks can be helpful in up to 75% of women.

Sacral neuromodulation is an invasive yet promising technique currently under investigation for treatment of refractory interstitial cystitis (62). In a small retrospective study, 21 patients with

Table 9. Multimodal Management of Interstitial Cystitis and Bladder Pain Syndrome

Class of Treatment	Medications or Interventions	Dose
Behavioral modification	Dietary restrictions (avoidance of spicy and acidic food)	
	Bladder training	
	Cognitive behavioral therapy	
	Stress management	
	Pelvic floor physical therapy (if coexisting hypertonic pelvic floor)	
Analgesic	Nonsteroidal anti-inflammatory drugs	Trial of usual dosages may be employed as first-line therapy
	Opioids	
Mucosal surface protection	Pentosan polysulfate (oral or intravesical)	100 mg, orally three times per day for 6 months
	Hyaluronic acid (intravesicular)	40 mg weekly for 6 weeks (under investigation)
	Heparin sulfate (subcutaneous or intravesical)	Self-administered three times per week for 3 months
	Chondroitin sulfate (oral)	Under investigation
Mast cell or histamine inhibition	Pentosan polysulfate and heparin	Self-administered three times per week for 3 months
	Hydroxyzine (H_1 receptor antagonist)	Under investigation
	Cimetidine (H_2 receptor antagonist)	Under investigation
Antidepressant therapy	Tricyclic antidepressant amitriptyline	10 mg, orally every night should be titrated to 150 mg
Nociceptive pathway desensitization	Dimethyl sulfoxide (intravesical)	Intravesical treatments every 1–2 weeks for 4–8 weeks, under investigation
	Lidocaine	
Surgical	Sacral neuromodulation	Under investigation

chronic pelvic pain attributed to refractory interstitial cystitis confirmed by cystoscopy and hydrodistention underwent implantation of a device aimed at sacral nerve root stimulation (63).

A total of 20 patients reported a moderate to marked decrease in pain and a 36% reduction in average daily narcotic dose. Subsequent small prospective studies also have shown significant improvement in pain scores with a greater than 50% reduction in pain and a 42% reduction in other symptoms. Sacral neuromodulation is not currently FDA approved for interstitial cystitis, and larger studies are required to confirm efficacy.

> **CASE NO. 3.** A 38-year old woman, gravida 2, para 2, is referred from her primary care physician with a 1-year history of pelvic pain. The pain is described as deep, achy, suprapubic pain, with a score of 4 out of 10 in severity, and worsening before and during the menstrual period. Menses are regular with normal flow and duration. The patient endorses a history of urinary frequency, urgency, nocturia, and mild deep dyspareunia. She does not have hematuria, hematochezia, constipation, or diarrhea. She has a past medical history significant for IBS and hypothyroidism, which are well controlled. She currently uses oral contraceptives and thyroid supplementation. Surgical history is positive for two cesarean deliveries. Physical examination reveals normal abdominal examination without trigger points, masses, or organomegaly; mild suprapubic tenderness of the external genitalia; and normal vaginal epithelium. Pelvic floor muscles are not tender but her ability to relax after a Kegel exercise is poor. The bimanual examination is normal with the exception of a tender bladder. There are no social or psychologic issues, and her relationship with her husband is excellent. Urinalysis, urine culture, cervical gonorrhea and chlamydia PCR testing, and transvaginal ultrasonography all yield normal results.

The differential diagnosis includes overactive bladder, IC/BPS, adenomyosis, endometriosis, and IBS flare. The new pain associated with irritative voiding symptoms is suggestive of IC/BPS. At this time, she does not associate pain with altered stool form or frequency, increase in pain before a bowel movement, and decrease after a bowel movement, making IBS an unlikely diagnosis. Her bimanual examination yielded normal results; she is parous and does not have a history of subfertility or prior endometriosis. Therefore, endometriosis is an unlikely diagnosis but should not be completely ruled out. Adenomyosis often results in a somewhat enlarged and tender uterus and may have some features of myometrial heterogeneity on ultrasonography. Usually, there is more dysmenorrhea and menorrhagia than in this case.

Evaluation included a KCl instillation test of which the result was positive, but in this case the diagnosis can be established clinically. The presence of pain argues against overactive bladder. Pelvic floor myofascial symptoms could account for pain, urinary symptoms, and dyspareunia. The patient started a diet to reduce overactive bladder, a trial of amitriptyline, 10 mg, increased to 50 mg at bedtime, and pelvic floor physical therapy. Bladder instillations with anesthetic solutions and pentosan polysulfate therapy can be added, if needed. This case illustrates that women with pain not related to the reproductive system often come to their gynecologist for care, and such patients can be treated by gynecologists or by urologists.

Vulvar and Perineal Pain

Vulvar Vestibulitis Syndrome or Vestibulodynia. Pain and hypersensitivity in the vestibule without physical findings other than allodynia (pain with gentle touch) and erythema are the most common cause of entry dyspareunia. Such condition is now called provoked (with touching) or unprovoked (spontaneous) localized vestibulodynia because biopsy specimens of patients who ultimately receive this diagnosis exhibit the same degree of inflammation on routine histology as control specimens.

Vestibulodynia is further categorized as primary (presenting on initiation of intercourse or first tampon use) or secondary (presenting after a period of normal response to intercourse). The etiology remains unclear; although several studies have attempted to elucidate a causative factor, results are conflicting. There are studies that show an association between candidiasis and other genital infections. Also, an allergic mechanism has been proposed as an etiology because levels of immunoglobulin E consistent with vaginal allergy have been found; antihistamines, however, have not proved effective. Others have suggested a genetic predisposition that impairs the immune system's ability to stop the reactive inflammatory response triggered by exposure to infection or chemicals. The affected tissue shows increased activity in nerve endings; increased levels of mast cells, nerve growth factor, and substance P; and immunohistochemical binding compared with controls, although histologic studies show no evidence of inflammation with leukocytes. Vestibulodynia often is associated with interstitial cystitis, which is commonly attributed either to shared embryologic origins of the bladder mucosa, vestibule, and urethra within the urogenital sinus or to cross-sensitization.

The diagnosis of vestibulodynia is one of exclusion. The patient's medical history usually will reveal entry dyspareunia and pain associated with insertion of tampons or even with the use of restrictive clothing. Diagnostic application of light pressure with a cotton swab on the vestibule produces extreme pain. The differential diagnosis is extensive and includes hypoestrogenism related to menopause, breastfeeding, use of low-dose hormonal contraception, candidiasis, herpes, allergic dermatitis, lichen sclerosis, lichen planus, or pudendal neuropathy. Wet mount test with saline solution and a potassium hydroxide test are useful to assess estrogenization (increase in parabasal and intermediate cells), vaginitis from yeast, trichomonas, desquamative inflammatory vaginitis, lichen planus, and bacterial vaginosis. Yeast cultures and vulvar or vaginal biopsy may be necessary. Pelvic floor muscle tightness and tenderness should be assessed and any tenderness along the pudendal nerve noted.

Treatment recommendations should include behavioral modification, ie, avoiding contact with irritative products and clothing. Tricyclic antidepressants are the first-line agents used for medical management of vestibulodynia. Amitriptyline, nortriptyline, and desipramine therapy (with amitriptyline being the most sedative and desipramine, the least sedating) should be started at the lowest dose of 10 mg and titrated up to an effective dose, but may require doses up to 75–100 mg nightly for improvement of symptoms. Local anesthetic is another mainstay of treatment. Topical lidocaine, 5%, in a nonirritating base should be used nightly and 20–30 minutes before intercourse to improve dyspa-

reunia. One double-blinded, four-arm placebo-controlled trial of
the TCA desipramine taken orally or lidocaine, 5%, applied topically at night to the vestibule, or a combination of both therapies,
failed to find a benefit compared with placebo (64). However,
because many of the patients in the study did respond well to
this combined therapy, the data are currently being analyzed to
determine which factors in the patients' histories predict a positive therapeutic response. Based on uncontrolled studies, anesthetics should be applied at least nightly and possibly up to three
times per day for cases of unprovoked constant pain. Gabapentin
administered nightly in a topical formulation (6% gabapentin
cream) was effective in an uncontrolled study. Second-line medical therapy includes oral anticonvulsants, such as gabapentin or
pregabalin, in patients who are intolerant to or unresponsive to
topical mediations or TCAs. Gabapentin, for example, is initiated at 100 mg nightly and increased by 100 mg every 2–7 days
titrated to a maximum of 3,600 mg daily in three to four divided
doses. Up to 120 mg can be administered at night if daytime
doses are too sedating. Pregabalin, a newer GABAergic agent,
can be used if gabapentin fails to bring relief. Up to 600 mg of
pregabalin can be administered daily in two to three divided
doses. Submucous infiltrations of lidocaine and methylpredniso-
lone acetate were useful in one study with complete remission in
seven of 22 women with vestibulodynia (65). Symptom improvement in 50% of patients has been observed in one uncontrolled
study with five biweekly sessions of 10 mL of 0.2% ropivacaine
through caudal epidural, 10 mL of 0.25% bupivacaine bilateral
pudendal nerve block, and 10 mL 0.25% bupivacaine vestibular
infiltration (66).

Vestibulodynia has been associated with vaginal hypertonicity,
decreased vaginal muscle strength, and restriction of the vaginal
opening. Pelvic floor physical therapy aimed at addressing these
issues results in improvement of symptoms. Vaginal dilators
can be used in an attempt to practice relaxation during penetration to overcome abnormal pelvic floor muscular responses.
Electromyography biofeedback and biofeedback-assisted pelvic
physical therapy also have been found to reduce pain in many
women. A 2001 study that compared group cognitive–behavioral
therapy, surface electromyography biofeedback, and vestibulec-

tomy, found that all three study groups experienced significant improvements in psychologic adjustment and sexual function, although surgical therapy was found to be superior (67).

Surgical therapy is an option for patients whose symptoms are refractory to medical management or who cannot tolerate the adverse effects of pharmacotherapy. One type is surgical excision of the vestibule (Woodruff procedure) in which the surgeon may map and excise the affected area and cover it with undermined vaginal epithelium. Many surgeons remove the entire vestibule to avoid the possibility of recurrence. A review of these surgical techniques revealed that there is significant variation with respect to surgical technique, and appropriate extent of excision is unknown (68). Up to 90% of women reported satisfaction with results, and abstention from intercourse decreased to less than 15% on average. Other studies suggest 50% of patients have a good response. Potential postoperative complications include poor healing, hematoma formation, infection, Bartholin gland obstruction, and in approximately 5% of patients, increased pain (69).

CASE NO. 4. A 68-year-old woman, gravida 1, para 1, presents with a 1-year history of vulvar pain. She describes the pain as burning with a score of 5 out of 10 in severity. The pain increases with sitting, tight clothing, and intercourse. For the past year, she has also had urinary frequency and urgency, but no incontinence. She has seen a urologist and received a diagnosis of irritable bladder. An anticholinergic drug was prescribed that helped her urinary symptoms minimally, but did not improve the pain. This patient has a lifelong history of constipation. She does not report any recent injury and she does not exercise. She initially thought she had a yeast infection, but this was ruled out and she was prescribed estrogen cream, which she has used three times per week for almost 1 year. Menopause occurred 10 years ago and she had never used hormonal medications before this year. Her sexual history was basically negative. She is married and has an excellent relationship with her husband and was sexually active without problems with libido, arousal, orgasm, or pain until last year. She admits to moderate anxiety, but denied symptoms of depression. Past medical history includes osteoarthritis. Her obstetric–gynecologic history is noncontributory. She has had one normal spontaneous vaginal delivery and no prior surgery. Her medications include ibuprofen and estrogen cream. Physical examination reveals a normal appearing vulva with the exception of moderate erythema of the vulvar vestibule. The cotton swab revealed tenderness that is limited to this area but no vulvar lesions or other areas of tenderness were found. Vagina is moist and pink, without discharge, pelvic relaxation, or lesions. Wet mount saline preparation and potassium chloride test results are normal and epithelial cells appear well estrogenized. Palpation of the levator ani muscles reveals tightness and tenderness of the iliococcygeus bilaterally. There is tenderness over Alcock canal bilaterally. The remainder of the pelvic examination is within normal limits without tenderness. The pain with intercourse is reproduced with vestibular and pelvic floor muscle palpation.

This patient has vulvodynia that is localized and generalized and provoked and unprovoked. The etiology is multifactorial and includes neuropathic, myofascial, and CNS factors. Constipation and anxiety are factors that contribute to and maintain the pain and must be addressed.

Management should be tailored to the patient's symptoms, past treatments, and her ability to tolerate the various adverse effects of the available pharmacologic agents. Pharmacotherapy includes nerve threshold altering medications, administered topically, orally, or both. Alternatively, if indicated, they can be administered by injection (ie, vulvar vestibular infiltration, pudendal nerve blocks, and if available, caudal epidural with local anesthetic agents). Lidocaine, 2–5%; gabapentin, 6% compound, or both applied nightly to the vulvar vestibule for 3–6 months is an appropriate first-line therapy. For this patient, oral TCA, SNRI, or an anticonvulsant starting with a low dose administered at night and increased as tolerated to an effective dose also would be useful. If this dose cannot be reached because of the effects or is not effective, another agent should be used.

Contributing symptoms should be assessed, such as anxiety (for a referral to a psychiatrist if medication is needed or a psychologist for cognitive–behavioral or relaxation therapy or hypnosis) and constipation (for treatment with diet modification and medication or for a possible referral to a gastroenterologist).

Physical therapy should be initiated to include pelvic floor muscles and other contributing myofascial factors. Sexual intimacy even if it does not include intercourse should be encouraged. The patient should be asked to keep a simple pain rating scale nightly to assess progress, call in if she cannot tolerate the medication as prescribed, and follow up every 3 months or sooner if nerve blocks are administered. Surgery (vestibulectomy) can be considered as a last resort if all other modalities fail to bring relief, pain is localized to the vestibule, and other factors have been treated.

Vulvodynia. The pathophysiology of vulvodynia remains unclear, but it may represent a type of pudendal neuropathy or other neuropathic neuroplastic pain disorder initiated by a wide variety of mechanisms, including compression, chronic inflammation, referred pain from IC/BPS, and even systemic conditions, such as multiple sclerosis and fibromyalgia or, in most cases, idiopathic causes.

The pudendal nerve innervates the labia majora and minora, clitoris, urethral meatus, vulvar vestibule, perineum, and perianal skin, and any of these areas may be affected. Patients often report stinging, burning, irritation, rawness or pain of the vulva that often occurs with sitting or after intercourse.

There are commonly no physical findings in patients with this disorder, and any suspicious findings on physical examination should prompt biopsy to rule out other etiologies. Physical examination reveals a lack of erythema, edema, white or red lesions, erosions, or fibrosis. If any skin changes are present, exclusion of infectious, dermatologic, neoplastic, or other diagnosis is warranted. Levator ani muscle contraction on examination may be suggestive of the myofascial contributions to the diagnosis. If tenderness is noted along the pudendal nerve, a pudendal block is useful for diagnosis as well as treatment because affected patients often feel relief for hours, days, or weeks after injection.

Pudendal blocks can be repeated up to five times, and can be performed with ultrasound or CT guidance for improved precision and safety. For severe pudendal entrapment in the Alcock canal, the pudendal nerve motor latency test result often will be abnormal.

Nonsteroidal antiinflammatory drugs and TCA therapy or anticonvulsants usually are used as first-line treatments; otherwise, the management is similar to that of vestibulodynia discussed earlier in this section. Nerve blocks also may be effective. For severe and refractory cases with abnormal pudendal nerve motor latency tests, surgical decompression of the pudendal canal can be considered. Cognitive–behavioral therapy and stress reduction are key elements as is pelvic floor physical therapy.

PERSISTENT GENITAL AROUSAL DISORDER

Formerly known as persistent sexual arousal syndrome, persistent genital arousal disorder is a condition that causes unwanted and unstimulated feelings of genital arousal, qualitatively different from sexual arousal that is preceded by sexual desire, subjective arousal, or both. Symptoms include engorgement, increased vaginal secretion, tingling, fullness, and painful spasms in the rectum and pelvic floor muscles, similar to orgasm. Most women find this condition distressing and report only brief relief with self-stimulation to orgasm. Preexisting anxiety and depression are common in this group of patients. Most women are relieved to learn they have a genital pain disorder and not a sexual disorder. The cause of this condition can be both medical and psychologic, but is essentially unknown. Case reports have documented this disorder after the discontinuation of SSRIs, particularly trazodone. Physical therapy, cognitive–behavioral therapy, antidepressants, anxiolytics, and caudal or pudendal blocks may help relieve pain in women who have this condition.

Pain of Nongynecologic Origin

Gynecologic disorders are not the only cause of pelvic pain. Similar symptoms can be caused by several different conditions, such as GI or musculoskeletal disorders. As a woman's primary health care provider, the obstetrician–gynecologist should be fairly comfortable in differentiating disorders of various etiologies and be familiar with the available diagnostic and therapeutic tools. At the same time, the obstetrician–gynecologist should be able to recognize when the referral to a specialist is necessary. Given the complex nature of many disorders, consultation or cotreatment of patients with pelvic pain is common. Ideally, the specialists and consultants, such as anesthesiologists, urologists, gastroenterologists, physical therapists, and psychotherapists, have experience in the diagnosis and management of chronic pain or pain disorders. A number of health care providers often become involved in the management of chronic pelvic pain in one patient, and care must be taken to ensure all health care providers are aware of the patient's current treatment regimen when initiating a new treatment plan. This demands consistent and detailed communication among all health care providers in order to maximize effectiveness and avoid adverse effects.

GASTROINTESTINAL DISORDERS

Gastrointestinal disorders are a common cause of chronic pelvic pain. The colon and reproductive organs share the same thoracolumbar and sacral autonomic and somatic innervations and thus have common regions of pain referral. Gastrointestinal disorders often coexist with gynecologic and myofascial pathologies because of viscerovisceral or viscerosomatic cross-sensitization whereby inflammation or infection in one organ can decrease the threshold for pain sensation in other pelvic organs and overlying muscle. Patients with GI symptoms may seek out or be referred to a gynecologist for multiple reasons, including pelvic pain disorders, premenstrual and menstrual exacerbation of GI pain, and GI symptoms related to gynecologic pathology (such as endometriosis).

Irritable Bowel Syndrome. Up to 60% of women referred to gynecologists for chronic pelvic pain are found to have IBS, which causes recurrent abdominal discomfort or pain associated with altered bowel habits (4). Abdominal pain usually is intermittent and crampy in the mid to lower quadrants. Symptoms usually worsen with eating, during periods of stress, anxiety, and depression, and with premenstrual and menstrual phases of the cycle. Irritable bowel syndrome can be categorized into three subgroups: 1) constipation dominant, 2) diarrhea dominant, and 3) with alternating bowel habits. Physical examination generally is normal.

The diagnosis of IBS has been standardized by the Rome III criteria. The Rome III criteria require the presence of recurrent abdominal pain or discomfort for at least 3 days per month during the previous 3 months. In addition, the pain must meet two of the following characteristics: 1) it must be relieved by defecation, 2) its onset is associated with change in stool frequency, or 3) its onset is associated with change in stool form or appearance. Other symptoms supporting the diagnosis of IBS include altered stool frequency, altered stool passage (straining, urgency, or both), mucorrhea, abdominal bloating, or subjective distention (70). Irritable bowel syndrome is a diagnosis of exclusion and other more serious conditions should be ruled out. Recommended evaluation includes complete blood count, stool occult blood testing, measurements of electrolyte and thyroid stimulating hormone levels, and often endoscopy. Patients with chronic diarrhea should be evaluated for IBS, celiac sprue, or acute infection.

Management of IBS is multidisciplinary and includes education and reassurance, dietary modification, stress reduction, and medical management. Given the psychologic component of this condition, the incorporation of cognitive–behavioral therapy is strongly advocated (71). Dietary changes often are helpful, particularly avoidance of lactose, sorbitol, alcohol, and caffeine. After a trial of diet modification and fiber supplementation, a short-term trial of an antispasmodic agent, such as dicyclomine or hyoscyamine, is appropriate for persistent symptoms.

Table 10 summarizes the pharmacologic management of IBS. Initial management involves treatment of constipation or diarrhea symptoms. Regular passage of stool in patients with constipation-predominant IBS may improve pain and bloating, whereas control of loose stools in diarrhea-predominant IBS will improve quality of life but typically have resulted in little change in pain symptoms. Tegaserod, a 5-HT_4 agonist, is approved by the FDA for women with constipation-predominant IBS. It has visceral and antinociceptive effects and is beneficial as a short-term treatment, but its use should be limited to patients younger than 55 years and without known ischemic CV risks. Antispasmodic agents function by relaxing the smooth muscle and reducing contractility of the GI tract. Serotonin receptor antagonists target 5-HT_3 receptors located on enteric nervous system sensory neurons. These

Table 10. Treatment of Irritable Bowel Syndrome

Medication Class	Mechanism	Dose
Tricyclic antidepressants	Modulate descending serotonergic and noradrenergic pain inhibition systems→decreased sensitivity to somatic pain	Amitriptyline, 10–75 mg nightly Nortriptyline, 10–75 mg nightly
	Have anticholinergic attributes→alter gastrointestinal motility	Desipramine, 50–150 mg nightly
Selective serotonin reuptake inhibitors	Serotonin receptor agonist ($5HT_2$) treats depression and anxiety, decreases abdominal pain and bloating, and improves overall well-being	Paroxetine, 10–60 mg daily Citalopram, 5–20 mg daily Fluoxetine, 20–40 mg daily
Serotonin norepinephrine receptor inhibitors	Affect descending serotonergic and noradrenergic pain inhibition systems	Duloxetine, 30–60 mg daily Milnacipran, 50–100 mg twice per day (titrated from 12.5 mg twice per day) Venlafaxine, 37.5–225 mg daily
Antidiarrheals	Slow gut motility	Loperamide, 2 mg daily
Other		
Alosetron	Serotonin receptor antagonist ($5HT_3$) decreases stool frequency and bowel urgency and relieves abdominal pain and discomfort	0.5–1mg twice per day
Tegaserod	Partial $5\text{-}HT_4$ agonist	6 mg twice per day
Hyoscyamine	Antispasmodic	Hyoscyamine, 0.125–0.25 mg four times per day Dicyclomine 10–20 mg four times per day Mebeverine, 135–200 mg four times per day

receptors are responsible for stimulation of intestinal motility. Serotonin receptor antagonists slow the rate of colonic transit and reduce gastrocolic reflex.

Antispasmodics and laxatives may produce symptomatic relief of bowel symptoms, and the pain symptoms of IBS may respond to antidepressants. Low-dose TCAs have been shown to relieve pain associated with IBS in a number of RCTs, with a meta-analysis reporting benefit of TCAs compared with placebo for improvement of pain (72). Pain reduction may be related to decreased sensitivity of peripheral nerves. Tricyclic antidepressants also are known to reduce excessive GI contractility and are approved for use as antispasmodics. Tricyclic antidepressants may be used in women with moderate to severe pain as a predominant symptom that is refractory to other therapies. Although high doses of antidepressants are not necessary to achieve the antinociceptive response, TCAs may be titrated up to high doses in patients with comorbid depression. Selective serotonin reuptake inhibitors and SNRIs also have been used successfully in the treatment of IBS and should be used in patients in whom TCA treatment has failed or those who are depressed or unable to tolerate the adverse effects of TCAs.

Functional Abdominal Pain Syndrome. Functional abdominal pain syndrome is estimated to occur in 0.5–2% of the population and has been associated with a decrease in quality of life and functionality. Abdominal pain associated with this condition typically is described by patients as intense, diffuse, and nonlocalized. The pain may be described in an emotional or bizarre fashion, and patients may request diagnostic studies or surgery; however, these patients may deny a psychosocial component of pain. Physical examination generally yields normal results.

Diagnosis is based on the presence of the following symptoms for at least 6 months and exclusion of any other GI disorder: 1) continuous or nearly continuous abdominal pain; 2) pain not typically associated with physiologic events, such as eating or menstrual bleeding, 3) loss of daily function, and 4) absence of malingering.

A multidisciplinary approach offers the most promise for improvement of symptoms. The key to treatment is a good physician–patient relationship with open communication and education regarding the diagnosis, management plan, and treatment goals. No valuable research regarding psychotherapeutic approaches in this disorder has been conducted to date. Antidepressants such, as TCAs or SSRIs, can alleviate symptoms.

Inflammatory Bowel Disease. Inflammatory bowel disease encompasses two main disorders: 1) ulcerative colitis and 2) Crohn disease, which are caused by abnormal activation of the mucosal immune system. These disorders are thought to result in pain through multiple mechanisms, including inflammation and obstruction, or from disease extension beyond the bowel wall (perforation, fistulization, or abscess formation). Crohn disease is more commonly associated with abdominal pain, stricture formation, and perirectal or perianal involvement. Symptoms are typically intermittent but chronic in both ulcerative colitis and Crohn disease. Abdominal pain is the most common symptom, affecting 82% of patients, followed by diarrhea (70%), weight loss (56%), and rectal bleeding (26%).

The initial presentation of inflammatory bowel disease usually involves abdominal pain and diarrhea with or without rectal bleeding. Because these symptoms may be nonspecific, patients must be systematically evaluated for other possible diagnoses, including infectious gastroenteritis, infection with *Clostridium difficile*, intestinal tuberculosis, diverticulitis, intestinal lymphoma, and cancer. Obtaining a thorough history plays an important role in evaluating a patient with pain symptoms and diarrhea. Stool studies for bacteria, ova, and parasites should be conducted to rule out infectious colitis. A definitive diagnosis is established with endoscopy of the upper and lower GI tracts. Barium enema studies should be avoided because they may cause ileus and subsequent toxic megacolon.

A diagnosis or suspicion of inflammatory bowel disease is an indication for referral to a gastroenterologist. Treatment of ulcerative colitis and Crohn disease is based on decreasing the chronic inflammation. Sulfasalazine or mesalamine are most commonly used as initial treatments. Corticosteroid use is limited to disease flares and other immunosuppressive agents, such as cyclosporine, methotrexate, and azathioprine, are reserved for refractory cases.

Endometriosis of the Gastrointestinal Tract. Endometriosis of the GI tract or enterocolic endometriosis (also known as bowel endometriosis) is almost always associated with genital organ and peritoneal endometriosis. Up to 37% of women with pelvic endometriosis have bowel endometriosis. Most cases of bowel endometriosis involve the sigmoid colon (65%); other sites include the rectum, ileum, cecum, appendix, and small bowel. Microscopically, there are endometriotic-like glands and stroma infiltrating the bowel wall through the subserosal tissue.

However, when the lesions involve only the serosa, it is called peritoneal endometriosis. In the muscularis layer of the bowel, endometriotic foci surrounded by submucosal hyperplasia and fibrosis can form nodules. Pain is a result of infiltration of the adjacent neurovascular branches. The differential diagnosis of bowel endometriosis is highly variable, depending on its presentation and location and includes IBS, inflammatory bowel disease, diverticulitis, functional abdominal pain and bloating syndrome, and GI or ovarian carcinoma. There are no definitive recommendations for the evaluation of patients with suspected endometriosis of the GI tract.

The most common symptoms are dysmenorrhea, chronic pelvic pain, dyspareunia, dyschezia, nausea, or bloating. Some women with lesions may experience no pain, whereas other women may have excruciating pain with severity of symptoms often depending on the size and location of the lesions. Symptoms overlap with those of IBS and endometriosis. Small nodules on serosal surfaces usually are asymptomatic; larger lesions in the lower colon can cause diarrhea, constipation, bloating, or pain. Nausea and bloating may be caused by a sympathetic response from severe visceral pain, as seen in IBS. Unlike IBS, defecation does not reduce symptoms. Cyclical rectal bleeding is rare. Patients also may have dyschezia, tenesmus, and even acute bowel obstruction.

Tender nodules reflecting indurations in the cul-de-sac usually are noted on rectovaginal examination. Definitive diagnosis can usually be established with laparoscopy. No imaging procedure has been established as a standard tool for visualizing bowel endometriosis. Transvaginal ultrasonography has a sensitivity and specificity of 95% and 100%, respectively. It may allow visualization of bowel endometriosis as an irregular hypoechoic mass with hypoechoic or hyperechoic foci that infiltrate the mucosa, but it is difficult to see lesions above the rectosigmoid junction. Rectal endoscopic ultrasonography evaluates the involvement of the muscularis layer of the bowel and depth of infiltration of lesions, with a sensitivity and specificity of 97.1% and 89.4%, respectively, but cannot visualize the upper colon and requires anesthesia, rendering it impractical in the office setting. Double contrast barium enema has been used since the 1980s for diagnosing bowel endometriosis, but the specificity of this test is low, visualizing only intrusions into the lumen, and it cannot assess the full thickness of the bowel wall or the depth of infiltration of the lesions. Colonoscopy is not particularly useful because most lesions do not penetrate the mucosa. The sensitivity and specificity of MRI are 76.5% and 97.9%, respectively. However, it is not possible to visualize a nodule located more than 8 cm above the anal margin.

Management of bowel endometriosis must take into account the severity of symptoms and the effect on quality of life. Expectant management is an option, as long as there are no signs of bowel obstruction. Medical therapies have been used with mixed results because most lesions are fibrotic. Surgery is recommended if there is pain or evidence of obstruction. Most studies examining postoperative outcomes are retrospective; complete relief (or near complete relief) is estimated to occur in 72–86% of patients after resection. The disease may recur in less than 5%; however, it is unclear just how much to resect and when to perform surgery if obstruction is absent. Most trials have shown a modest improvement in pain and quality of life.

Colorectal Cancer. Colorectal cancer is the second most common cause of cancer-related death in the United States. It usually occurs in women older than 45 years. Box 7 summarizes the warning signs of colorectal cancer.

Box 7. Risk Factors and Warning Signs of Colorectal Cancer

- Age older than 50 years
- Personal and family history of colon cancer or certain types of colon polyps
- Tarry stools
- Blood in stools
- Weight loss
- Severe diarrhea

Despite advances in screening, most cases are still diagnosed clinically. The most common symptoms are rectal bleeding, hematochezia, and vague abdominal pain, which may predominate on the side of the lesion. These symptoms often are similar to those of benign conditions. Rectal bleeding, for example, occurs in 3–15% of the population. However, colorectal cancer is diagnosed in only 3% of these patients. Other symptoms, such as abdominal pain and changes in bowel habits also are common in other benign conditions, such as IBS. Symptoms common with proximal cancer may include anemia, anorexia, nausea, vomiting, and abdominal pain, whereas distal tumors are commonly associated with rectal bleeding, altered stools, rectal pain, or tenesmus. Patients typically report symptoms that last more than 6 weeks, and may report constitutional symptoms, such as fatigue, weight loss, and night sweats.

Fecal occult blood testing can be ordered as a screening test, particularly in women with anemia of unclear etiology. However, a positive fecal occult blood test result is present in 75% of asymptomatic individuals. Patients in whom colorectal cancer is suspected should undergo endoscopic evaluation because most lesions arise from the mucosa. Colonoscopy is considered the standard diagnostic test because it allows visualization of the entire colon and facilitates biopsy.

A diagnosis of cancer requires referral to a surgical oncology specialist for appropriate staging and treatment planning. Further discussion of specific surgical and nonsurgical management is beyond the scope of this monograph.

Hernia. Hernias are uncommon in women. However, if one is encountered on examination and reproduces the pain, it should be included on the differential evaluation. Symptoms and signs include abdominal pain, mass, or both and pain or discomfort with increased intraabdominal pressure (Table 11). If a hernia is suspected, referral to a general surgeon is recommended.

Musculoskeletal Disorders

One of the most commonly overlooked regions in the evaluation of chronic pelvic pain is the musculoskeletal system. Careful evaluation of the abdominal wall, low back, and pelvic floor muscles

Table 11. Hernia and Pelvic Pain

Type	Incidence	Location	Signs
Direct inguinal	25% of all hernias	Defect of weakness of transversalis fascia of Hesselbach triangle (bounded by inguinal ligament, inferior epigastric arteries, and conjoined tendon)	Inguinal bulge
Indirect inguinal	50% of all hernias; occurs at any age	Follows gastrointestinal tract through the inguinal ligament	Inguinal bulge
Femoral	3% of hernias (mostly in females)	Below the inguinal ligament through the femoral canal	Bulge below inguinal ligament and medial thigh pain, groin pain, or both
Umbilical	More common in males	Involves the umbilical fibromuscular ring, which usually obliterates by age 2 years	Bulge in umbilical area
Incisional or ventral	10% of all hernias	At incision site	Increase in size with standing or increased intra-abdominal pressure
Spigelian	Rare	Lateral to the rectus muscle at the semilunar line (costal arch to pubic tubercle)	Bulge lateral to rectus muscle
Obturator	Rare, but mostly occurs in women (women-to-men ratio of 6:1)	Through obturator foramen	Obstructive symptoms, medial thigh pain, and weight loss

can be readily accomplished at the time of the abdominal and pelvic examinations.

Myofascial Pain Syndrome. Myofascial pain disorders are distinguished by localized tenderness and pain in soft tissues, most commonly the back, head, and shoulders, but pain in the abdominal wall and that in the pelvic floor also are well recognized. The prevalence of myofascial pain in general is widely varied (15–89%) and may account for up to 30% of pain-related diagnoses in an internal medicine practice. These disorders are commonly associated with other pain syndromes, such as fibromyalgia. Myofascial pain syndrome is diagnosed in 30% of patients with regional pain who go to primary care clinics and 85% who go to pain centers. It is a condition caused by trigger points in muscle or muscle fascia. A trigger point is an area of hyperirritability and tenderness in a taut, palpable band of muscle fibers (73).

Myofascial pain syndrome can be classified into two stages: 1) in the initial neuromuscular stage, fiber injury and subsequent release of neurotransmitters, inflammatory mediators, and immune chemotaxis result in overactivity of afferent nociceptors and development of new trigger points by way of central sensitization; 2) the second stage, termed musculodystrophic, results from prolonged contractile activity that produces sustained release of noxious products and ultimately results in muscle fibrosis. Associated factors include chronic stress, anxiety, hypothyroidism, and malnutrition (74). Because of the aforementioned complex innervations of the pelvic structures, muscles (such as the rectus, iliopsoas, quadratus lumborum, piriformis, and obturator internus innervated through T-12–L-4, and levator ani, innervated through S-2–S-3) can develop trigger points or tender points referred from the pelvic viscera.

Patients usually report dull aching or sharp stabbing pain that may be difficult to characterize. Exacerbation of pain in association with irritation either from pelvic pathology or menses and intercourse is common.

Lack of objective findings often hampers diagnosis. Digital examination may reveal tenderness to palpation, trigger points, or both that evoke local and referred pain. The bilateral straight leg-raising maneuver that tenses the abdominal wall muscles exacerbates abdominal wall pain.

The most important steps in the management of myofascial pelvic pain disorder are to determine whether there is a coexisting hypertonic pelvic floor disorder, and if so, to identify the underlying cause. Physical therapy and local anesthetic trigger point injections are the mainstay in the management of myofascial pain (73, 74). Physical therapy involves retraining the pelvic floor muscles with the use of biofeedback techniques, relaxation

techniques, and reverse Kegel exercises. If physical therapy fails
to alleviate persistent myofascial pelvic floor pain or abdominal
wall pain, trigger point injection therapy may be added to the
management regimen. A series of three to five injections may be
administered, which has been shown to provide sustained relief
for several weeks. Digital palpation is used to identify the trigger
point. The insertion of a 21- to 25-gauge needle into the palpable
trigger point may reproduce the patient's pain and may elicit a
muscle twitch. Local anesthetic is used to infiltrate the area followed by slightly withdrawing and readvancing into the trigger
point and its associated muscle band several times. The addition
of corticosteroids into the area is advocated by some experts, but
RCTs have not confirmed added benefit. A single 60-patient RCT
that compared lidocaine patch and placebo patch versus anesthetic injection for the treatment of myofascial pain syndrome
revealed similar efficacy of anesthetic patch and trigger point
injection, but the use of anesthetic patch was associated with less
discomfort than injection therapy (73). Psychologic factors, such
as stress, depression, anxiety, and maladaptive behavior should
be identified and treated. Medications, such as low-dose TCAs
and anticonvulsants also may be useful.

Pelvic Floor Spasm and Hypertonic Muscle Disorders.
Chronic pelvic pain syndromes, particularly vulvodynia and
IC/BPS, as well as colorectal pain disorders, such as proctalgia
fugax, anodynia, and IBS, often are associated with pelvic floor
muscle spasm and nerve irritation. The viscerosomatic reflex
and referred pain will trigger muscle spasm and myalgia in
the levator ani muscles, and the muscle contraction on nerve
branches running through the muscle will cause neuropathic
pain as well. Clinical syndromes associated with pelvic floor
hypertonic dysfunction or dyssynergia include childhood and
adulthood eliminating disorders, idiopathic urinary retention or
urgency frequency syndrome, constipation, anal incontinence,
and vaginismus.

   A history of dyspareunia, postcoital ache, and pain with sitting
are common. Patients will be unable to perform an adequate
Kegel exercise or to relax appropriately. Contracted, painful levator ani muscles (pubococcygeus, iliococcygeus, or coccygeus) are
found on examination (74).

Although there are no specific criteria for diagnosis, hyper-tonic or tender pelvic floor muscles on physical examination are highly suggestive of pelvic floor spasm and myalgia.

Management of any suspected underlying genital pain syndrome is important. Standard medical treatments, including TCAs and anticonvulsants, as discussed later can be helpful. Physical therapy is the treatment of choice. In one trial, 48 patients with a urologic pain syndrome were randomized to myofacial physical therapy or global therapeutic massage. Myofascial physical therapy was found to result in significant reduction in pain compared with massage therapy (75).

The use of botulinum toxin type A has been reported in a small double-blinded RCT. Although patients in both treatment and placebo groups experienced reduction in pain and dyspareunia, the patients in the botulinum group demonstrated significant reductions in pelvic floor pressure as measured by vaginal manometry compared with patients in the placebo group (76). Cognitive–behavioral therapy is an important adjunct. Sacral neuromodulation is particularly useful for refractory urinary urgency and anal pain syndromes.

Piriformis Syndrome. The piriformis muscle can compress or irritate the sciatic nerve, causing pain in the buttocks, perirectal area, and vulva and refer pain in the dermatome of the sciatic nerves L-4, L-5, and S-2–S-4 in a sciatica-like pattern down the back of the thigh to the bottom of the foot and even into the lower back. The piriformis muscle lies deep to the gluteal muscles, originating from the sacrum and attaching to the greater trochanter. The sciatic nerve generally passes beneath the piriformis muscle, but in 15% of individuals, it travels through the muscle itself where it is vulnerable if there is any chronic muscle injury that causes swelling of the muscle. The pain is increased by activities, such as biking, sitting, hip lateral rotation, leg abduction and hyperextension, and climbing stairs.

The diagnosis is based on symptoms and examination, but MRI and nerve conduction tests may be necessary to exclude lumbar disc herniation, hamstring tendonitis, and adhesions of other muscles around the sciatic nerve.

Treatment basically involves physical therapy that includes piriformis stretches. Injections of corticosteroid into the piriformis muscle and surgical exploration may be undertaken as second- and third-line therapy.

Fibromyalgia. Fibromyalgia is a chronic widespread pain syndrome of unclear etiology characterized by pain, fatigue, and mood and sleep disturbances. The disorder typically presents between the ages of 30 years and 55 years and is six times more common in females than in males. In approximately 50% of cases, the onset of symptoms seems to be associated with a specific event, such as a flu-like illness or even a traumatic emotional event.

The fundamental symptom of fibromyalgia is chronic and persistent musculoskeletal pain that usually involves several muscle groups in a symmetric fashion. The pain often is initially localized to the neck, back, and shoulders with eventual involvement of other muscle groups. Pain symptoms often are aggravated by stress, fatigue, and weather changes. Patients may report the sensation of joint swelling, but no evidence of joint inflammation will be detected on examination or imaging. Other sensations of dizziness, weakness, poor balance, numbness, and burning also can be reported. Fatigue is present in more than 90% of patients and may even be the original symptom. Abnormal sleep patterns include a spectrum of light sleep to sleep apnea. Most patients experience mood disturbances, such as depression and anxiety, and some even report cognitive dysfunction. The lifetime prevalence of depression in patients with fibromyalgia approaches 75%.

On physical examination, palpation of soft tissues reveals predefined "tender points," which are typically bilaterally symmetric (Box 8). Fibromyalgia is largely a diagnosis of exclusion. It is based primarily on the patient's history as described earlier. A comprehensive physical examination is performed and includes a complete rheumatologic examination to exclude arthritis, connective tissue disorders, or neurologic conditions. An examination of the nine pairs of tender points as described earlier also is performed as is the examination of some control areas (such as mid-arm or thigh). The examiner should apply pressure to those areas for several seconds using enough pressure to whiten the examiner's finger beds. The exact number of tender points to be used for diagnosis is not entirely clear but the current criteria, recommended by the American College of Rheumatology, include

> **Box 8. Fibromyalgia Tender Points**
>
> - Under lower sternomastoid muscle
> - Middle–upper trapezius muscle
> - Prominence of greater trochanter
> - Near second costochondral junction
> - Origin of supraspinatus muscle
> - Upper outer quadrant of buttock
> - Insertion of suboccipital muscle
> - Area 2 cm lateral to lateral epicondyle
> - Medial fat pad of the knee

the finding of tenderness in at least 11 of the 18 tender points, although this is mainly for research purposes. Patients also may undergo significant laboratory testing during the workup of their symptoms, including erythrocyte sedimentation rate measurement, thyroid function tests, and muscle enzymes, all of which yield negative results.

Because most patients with fibromyalgia have had the symptoms for years before an appropriate diagnosis was established and often worried that they had a serious underlying condition, confirming the diagnosis of fibromyalgia may be beneficial. Appropriate patient education is paramount and has been shown to both improve some of the mood symptoms associated with the disorder and decrease the number of further referrals and diagnostic testing. It can even result in a decrease in medication prescription and use. Patients should be reassured that although fibromyalgia is a real disorder, it is completely benign. Education about relaxation techniques, stress reduction, and exercise programs should be discussed with these patients because the symptoms are exacerbated by stress and immobility (77).

Antidepressants and anticonvulsants are the most commonly prescribed medications for fibromyalgia. Traditionally, TCAs, SSRIs, and SNRIs have been used and studied. Research has demonstrated that antidepressants are efficacious in the management of pain, fatigue, mood, and sleep symptoms as well as an improvement in health-related quality of life. The U.S. Food and Drug Administration has approved three drugs for the treatment of fibromyalgia: 1) duloxetine, 2) milnacipran, and 3) pregabalin. Tricyclic antidepressants have long been studied for the treatment of chronic pain disorders as discussed throughout this monograph. Trials of TCAs for the treatment of fibromyalgia have shown improvement in 24–45% of patients with the typically studied doses of amitriptyline, 25–50 mg nightly (78). Adverse effects are the limiting factors. Given the absence of tissue, muscle, or joint inflammation in patients with fibromyalgia, antiinflammatory medications, such as NSAIDs or prednisone, have been found to be no more effective than placebo for improvement of symptoms.

Neuropathic Causes of Pelvic Pain

Injury to or entrapment of the nerves of the anterior and lateral abdominal way, back, or vagina may result in chronic lower abdominal and perineal pain and dyspareunia. These nerves include the ilioinguinal nerve (T-12 and L-1), iliohypogastric nerve (T-12 and L-1), genitofemoral nerve (L-1 and L-2), pudendal nerve (S-2–S-4), and branches of the sciatic nerve (S-2–S-4). Injuries to these nerves may result in chronic lower abdominal and perineal pain. Low transverse skin incision, improper retractor positioning, improper lithotomy positioning, and radical surgical dissection during surgery are the most common causes of injury to sciatic nerve or abdominal wall nerves.

Pudendal neuropathy can result from vaginal surgery, especially with lateral mesh attachments, childbirth, and even chronic constipation or pelvic floor muscle abnormalities. Branches of the pudendal nerve, such as the vestibular, rectal, or clitoral branch, can be individually injured with vulvar surgical procedures, including episiotomy, laser hair removal, and Bartholin gland removal. The piriformis muscle can compress branches of the sciatic nerve, as noted, especially S-2, leading to lateral perirectal and perineal pain.

Stabbing, sharp, lancinating, or burning pain exacerbated by activity and chronic dull aching pain relieved by rest are com-

mon. Hyperesthesia and dysesthesia in areas of inner
common. Entrapment of the ilioinguinal or iliohypogastric
leads to pain at the lateral edge of the rectus margin and can
radiate to the hip, sacroiliac joint, or vulva. Pudendal neuropathy
causes burning, lancinating, or aching pain and allodynia in the
vulvar and perineal regions.

Physical examination detects focal tenderness to palpation over the site of nerve entrapment. For the examination of
the iliohypogastric and ilioinguinal nerves, the patient should
assume the supine position and the physician should palpate
the course of the suspected nerve, with a focus on regions of
suspected entrapment, generally 2–4 cm above the symphysis.
The examination should then be repeated with the patient tens-
ing her abdominal muscles (by extending and raising both legs
concurrently [straight leg raise or Carnet test] or by performing
an "abdominal crunch" maneuver). Palpation of the site with
muscles tensed reveals that the pain is worse. Pudendal nerve
pain is localized to the nerve distribution and the course of the
nerve is the area of maximal tenderness. Pudendal neuropathy is
described as consistent vulvar burning in the absence of physical
findings. Pudendal canal syndrome refers to the compression or
stretching of the pudendal nerve in the Alcock canal. The stretching caused by pudendal canal syndrome may be associated with
prolonged sitting, chronic straining attributed to constipation, or
after surgery or vaginal delivery.

Peripheral nerve blocks often are effective in relieving pain
and are both diagnostic and therapeutic. Bupivacaine, 0.25%,
or other local anesthetic agent is used for this purpose. Approximately 5 mL of the agent is injected into the point of maximal
tenderness with a 22–26 gauge, 1.5-inch needle. The needle
should slowly penetrate the subcutaneous tissue until the needle
tip reproduces the pain (79). Up to five biweekly injections
may be needed for improvement of symptoms. Direct injection
into the nerve (electrical sensation with needling) should be
avoided. Topical anesthetic creams or patches, low-dose TCAs,
anticonvulsants, and acupuncture are other options that may
improve symptoms (80). Nonsteroidal antiinflammatory drugs
and application of heat are helpful. Narcotic medications rarely
are completely effective. Long-term management of refractory

or recurrent cases includes cryoneurolysis or radio frequency ablation for abdominal wall neuropathies and neurolysis for certain cases of entrapment of abdominal wall nerves or pudendal nerves. Pudendal and sciatic neuropathies benefit from pelvic floor muscle physical therapy.

Psychosocial Contributors

It has been well established that chronic pain syndromes frequently are associated with depressive disorders, anxiety, and somatoform pain disorders. Malingering and substance abuse disorders also can occur. Psychosocial factors also play an important role in the perpetuation of chronic pain syndromes. Mental health professionals should be consulted if these factors are present.

Anxiety disorders that occur frequently in patients with chronic pain include generalized anxiety disorder, panic disorder, and posttraumatic stress disorder. Panic disorder criteria include the presence of recurrent unexplained panic attacks followed by at least a 1-month period of concern about having repeated attacks. A panic attack is a period of intense fear or discomfort associated with four of 13 symptoms, including chest pain, rapid heartbeat, diaphoresis, shortness of breath, nausea or abdominal discomfort, and paresthesias.

Somatization disorders consist of pain in four or more body parts or organs, one GU and two GI symptoms other than pain, and a neurologic symptom without pathology, such as weakness, dizziness, paralysis, or vision changes.

Substance abuse is difficult to diagnose in patients with chronic pain because many will be prescribed narcotics for severe pain and may develop physical tolerance and even unusual hoarding and illicit behavior ("pseudoaddiction"), if they are denied adequate narcotic pain relief. However, they may have a maladaptive pattern of substance use interfering with recreational and occupational activities or use of substances in larger amounts or for longer durations than normally intended. In one study of patients who received narcotics for chronic pain, nearly 25% of these patients developed narcotic addiction (dependence and abuse) over 3 years of treatment (81), but in another study, only 12% of patients with chronic pain were found to have psychologic dependency on analgesics (82). Patients who received opioids or benzodiazepines for acute or end-of-life pain or anxiety or sleep disorders were unlikely to develop psychologic dependence.

Suicidal potential is increased because of chronic pain, depression, and impulsivity and substance abuse or dependence. Patients should be asked if they have thought of ending their lives and especially if they have thought of specific ways to end their lives. Past attempts and family history of suicide increase the concern.

Nonspecific Chronic Pelvic Pain

Nonspecific pelvic pain is a term applied to a situation where no recognizable pain generator can be identified. It should not be a diagnosis of choice, but can be applied as a diagnosis of exclusion after a thorough history, physical examination, psychologic evaluation, and ancillary laboratory, imaging, or surgical investigations fail to find specific abnormalities. Invariably, in these cases, some degree of central sensitization has occurred. Nonspecific pharmacologic and nonpharmacologic approaches often are very helpful in these cases. Review of the pain ratings and triggers for pain usually will demonstrate stress and certain physical activities increase the pain. Cognitive–behavioral pain management or meditation, relaxation, and hypnosis as well as physical therapy are indicated. Many patients will want to try other CAM approaches. Depending on the findings of a physical examination, surgery may be helpful. For example, a tender uterus could indicate a neurectomy or hysterectomy, with the caveat that ancillary treatment may be necessary if pain persists.

PHARMACOLOGIC MANAGEMENT

Nonsteroidal antiinflammatory drugs function as prostaglandin inhibitors and also may mediate cytokines at the local level. Clinical evidence suggests that these drugs are very effective as first-line agents.

The role of opioid therapy in chronic pain remains controversial and RCTs are lacking. Long-term management of chronic pelvic pain with narcotic medications typically is considered as a last resort after failure of all other treatment modalities. Opioids should be given on a scheduled basis and should involve consistent follow-up with reassessments of the extent of pain relief, level of function, and quality of life. Physicians should ensure meticulous documentation of failure of other treatment options and patient counseling. The patient should sign a written narcotic contract agreeing to obtain pain medications from only one provider and delineating other expectations with respect to treatment (see the section "Special Considerations for Medication Management").

Tricyclic antidepressants and SNRIs have not been well studied for the treatment of chronic pelvic pain. Tricyclic antidepressants have shown efficacy in the treatment of many pain syndromes with a neuropathic or neuroplastic component. They are thought to improve pain tolerance, restore normal sleep patterns, and reduce depressive symptoms. Tricyclic antidepressants are initiated with the lowest doses (amitriptyline, 10 mg; nortripthyline, 10 mg; or desimipramine, 10 mg) and titrated up to 50–75 mg daily (Table 12). Full benefit may require at least 4 weeks of treatment. More data are needed to evaluate the effi-

Table 12. Doses of Antidepressants for Chronic Pain

Drug	Oral Dose Range (mg)	Anticholinergic Potency	Orthostatic Hypotension	Sedation
Tricyclic Antidepressants				
Amitriptyline	10–300	High	Moderate	High
Nortriptyline	50–150	Moderate	Low	Moderate
Desipramine	25–300	Low	Low	Low
Imipramine	20–300	High	High	Moderate
Selective Serotonin Reuptake Inhibitors				
Fluoxetine	5–40	None	None	None
Paroxetine	20–40	Low	None	None
Serotonin–Norepinephrine Reuptake Inhibitors				
Venlafaxine	37.5–300	None	None	None
Duloxetine	20–60	None	None	None

cacy of TCAs in the management of chronic pelvic pain specifically. In one small study, 14 women with chronic pelvic pain
who received negative laparoscopic results were treated with
nortriptyline, 50 mg daily. One half of these women dropped out
because of adverse effects. In the remaining seven patients, the
doses of nortriptyline were increased to 100 mg daily. Of these
patients, six were pain-free at a 1-year follow-up (3). Selective
serotonin reuptake inhibitors used for the treatment of chronic
pelvic pain have been studied in a single RCT that found no
significant difference in pain and functional status between the
users of sertraline and the users of placebo (83).

As previously discussed, gabapentin is now approved for use
in postherpetic neuralgia and has been shown to be successful in
the treatment of other neuropathic pain syndromes. Gabapentin
alone or in combination with amitriptyline was better than amitriptyline alone in a trial that compared 56 women with chronic
pelvic pain randomized to either gabapentin alone, amitriptyline
alone, or combination therapy with both drugs. At 6-, 12-, and
24-month follow-up visits, pain relief measured by visual analog
score was significantly improved in patients receiving gabapentin
either alone or in combination with amitriptyline compared with
patients receiving monotherapy with amitriptyline (84).

Loss of nociception also can be achieved locally by modalities,
such as trigger point injections or application of the botulinum
toxin type A. There are no RCTs specifically evaluating trigger
point injections in the management of chronic pelvic pain. In an
open label study of 122 women with chronic pelvic pain, abdominal wall trigger points were found in 89% of patients, vaginal
trigger points in 71% of patients, and sacral trigger points in 25%
of patients (85). Of these patients with trigger points, 52% were
pain free after a series of local anesthetic injections of the trigger
points. In a small uncontrolled prospective study of women with
chronic pelvic pain and levator ani muscle trigger points, patients
were treated with 10 mL of 0.25% bupivacaine, 10 mL of 2%
lidocaine, and 1 mL triamcinolone injected in 4-mL increments
into the trigger points (86). At a 3-month follow-up, 72% of
patients noted improvement in pain, and 33% of patients were
completely pain free.

Two case reports published in 2004 and 2005 reported improvement in pain and quality of life in a total of three women with chronic pelvic pain and levator ani spasm after injection of botulinum toxin type A (87, 88). This agent has analgesic properties for neuropathic pain and also may help by relieving muscle spasm. A subsequent double-blinded placebo controlled trial randomized 60 women with chronic pelvic pain and evidence of pelvic floor myalgia diagnosed by painful contracted muscles on palpation and elevated resting pressures (less than 40 cm H_2O) on vaginal manometry to injection of botulinum toxin type A versus placebo (76). Women treated with botulinum showed significant decrease in pressure as measured by vaginal manometry, decrease in pelvic floor muscle spasms, and improvement of symptoms of certain types of pelvic pain. However, improvements also were noted in the placebo group suggesting there is benefit to the act of simply disturbing the muscle with the needle. There was no difference in adverse outcomes between the two groups.

NONPHARMACOLOGIC MANAGEMENT

Physical Therapy. Physical therapy has been studied as a treatment modality for chronic pelvic pain. Given the association between many syndromes of chronic pelvic pain and hypertonic pelvic floor disorders, pelvic floor rehabilitation may play an important role in pain management. This therapy often begins with patient education because many of these women do not have awareness of the tension in their pelvic floor. Patients may have developed learned risk behaviors, such as holding urine, which should be eliminated. Awareness and retraining of these muscles can be taught through the use of biofeedback conducted by specially trained physical therapists.

Surgery. Large RCTs of various surgical procedures for the management of chronic pelvic pain are relatively few but are very important because of the high placebo effect associated with surgical intervention. The utility of laparoscopy in the diagnosis and management of chronic pelvic pain is somewhat controversial. Randomized controlled trials have not been performed because of the difficulty in randomization of surgical patients, variation in surgical techniques, and coexisting pain conditions (89). Nonsurgical therapy often is effective, is less costly, and has fewer risks than surgery. In fact, nonsurgical therapy is effective in 65–90% of patients regardless of pathology (90). A randomized trial compared laparoscopy with an integrated approach without laparoscopy that included assessment of somatic, psychologic, dietary, environmental, and physiotherapeutic factors. The integrated approach was significantly more effective in improving pelvic pain than laparoscopy alone; 75% versus 41%. Although an abnormal pelvic examination is associated with a 70–90% chance of pathology, almost one half of patients who receive normal results from preoperative pelvic examinations will have pathologic findings on laparoscopy. However, adhesions may not warrant adhesiolysis, and many women with endometriosis will respond to therapy with hormonal contraceptives. Additionally, even though the pathology is visualized, it may not be the cause of the patient's pain. Two thirds of patients have adhesions noted on laparoscopy that may or may not be associated with their chronic symptoms. Small endometriotic lesions may be physiologic and may regress without therapy. In general, laparoscopy should be reserved for carefully selected patients. General guidelines for selection include 1) patients in whom medication (hormonal and analgesic) has failed to relieve pain over a minimum of 3 months; 2) patients in whom endometriosis, hernias, and possibly adhesions have been managed surgically; 3) patients in whom associated infertility has been evaluated and managed.

Presacral neurectomy and laparoscopic uterosacral nerve ablation are surgical techniques that interrupt the neural input from the uterus. Sensory innervation of the reproductive organs is provided by the superior hypogastric plexus or presacral nerve (derived from T-11–T-12), pelvic nerves (S-2–S-4), and ovarian plexus (T-8–T-9). These sensory fibers from the uterus travel with sympathetic fibers entering the superior hypogastric plexus that consists of nerve bundles overlying L-4 to the promontory of sacrum. Presacral neurectomy refers to the transection of the pelvic thoracolumbar sympathetic autonomic innervation by removal of the presacral nerves lying within the boundaries of the interiliac triangle. Pain from the uterus can be obliterated, but pain from lateral structures is not affected by the presacral

neurectomy. Both sympathetic and parasympathetic fibers from
the uterus run in and around the uterosacral folds to the cervix.
Laparoscopic uterosacral nerve ablation refers to transection of
the uterosacral ligaments proximal to the uterine plexus, typically
at their insertion into the cervix. Presacral neurectomy, especially
one performed by laparoscopy, is technically more challenging
than laparoscopic uterine nerve ablation because of the proximity of the sacral vessels and right ureter. A randomized controlled
trial that compared 487 women who underwent laparoscopic
uterine nerve ablation versus those who underwent laparoscopy
alone yielded similar results without significant differences in
pain, dysmenorrhea, dyspareunia, or quality of life between the
two groups (91). The three RCTs of presacral neurectomy in
women with endometriosis have yielded inconsistent results.
The first two studies were small (92, 93). The most recent RCT,
which involved 63 women in each treatment group, studied the
division of the autonomic nerve at the presacral region along
with uterosacral ligament division compared with uterosacral
ligament division alone (94). This study did show a significant
improvement in dysmenorrhea, dyspareunia, and quality of life
in the women in the presacral neurectomy group. However,
additional RCTs are needed in this area of research. The most
common adverse effect is constipation (95). Studies that compare
uterosacral nerve ablation with presacral neurectomy have been
inconclusive. For example, in a review of nine RCTs (773 women)
that evaluated the efficacy of presacral neurectomy or uterosacral nerve ablation or compared the two modalities, results were
studied in a pooled analysis using pain relief as the primary outcome (96). This meta-analysis reported that laparoscopic uterine
nerve ablation was better than a control treatment, but presacral
neurectomy was more efficacious than laparoscopic uterine nerve
ablation for the management of primary dysmenorrhea. For the
management of secondary dysmenorrhea, presacral neurectomy
demonstrated significant improvement in pain symptoms at a
follow-up, whereas laparoscopic uterine nerve ablation conferred
no benefit compared with the control treatment.

It has been shown that 10–18% of hysterectomies are performed
for chronic pelvic pain, and self-reported satisfaction scores are
high among women who undergo hysterectomy for pain. How-

ever, definitive surgical management with hysterectomy remains controversial. The Maine Women's Health Study, a prospective cohort study, compared outcomes of 199 women with frequent pain at baseline. In this cohort, only 11% of women reported persistent symptoms after hysterectomy. Significant improvements also were noted in sexual function and psychologic symptoms (97). A retrospective study that evaluated 279 patients who underwent hysterectomy for chronic pelvic pain that lasted at least 6 months demonstrated that 74% of patients reported no pain, 21% of patients reported decreased pain, and 5% of patients reported unchanged or increased pain (98). Among women without identifiable pelvic disease, only 62% of patients reported resolution of pain at a 12-month follow-up. However, most of these studies were poorly controlled. Although many studies seem to indicate that hysterectomy may improve pain symptoms, the procedure is still controversial, particularly in young women and in women without obvious pelvic pathology. The decision to consider definitive surgical management should be made only after a careful preoperative evaluation and detailed patient counseling, including determining the risk-to-benefit ratio.

 Complementary and Alternative Medicine

Many women with chronic pelvic pain will seek nonconventional treatments either primarily or after failure of traditional medical management. It is vital to obtain a complete list of all therapies, medications, and supplements that the patient has used because of the potential for adverse interactions with other medications, including analgesics. For example, decreased seizure threshold has been reported during the concurrent use of anticonvulsants and certain herbal supplements, such as borage or evening primrose oil (99).

Few CAM approaches for the treatment of chronic pelvic pain have been subjected to RCTs, but some have extensive clinical support in the management of low back pain, arthritis, or other neuropathic or myofascial disorders and can be incorporated into the treatment plan. Because of the close relationship between

mood, stress, anxiety and chronic pain, many CAM modalities
may be successful treatment adjuncts in the multidisciplinary
approach.

Biologically based therapies are frequently marketed for the
treatment of a number of pelvic pain conditions, such as dysmenorrhea, IBS, IC/BPS, and other pain disorders. Vitamin B_6, evening primrose oil, calcium, and many others have been studied
most commonly in the setting of dysmenorrhea. The studies
evaluating the efficacy of these agents in reducing symptoms are
lacking or limited and underpowered, but most report benign
adverse effect profiles (100). Supplementation with omega-3 fatty
acids has been shown to improve pain symptoms and decrease
the amount of analgesics used in patients with certain inflammatory pain syndromes, such as rheumatoid arthritis. Although
further investigation is necessary to confirm their benefit in the
treatment of pelvic pain, these supplements generally have been
found to be safe (101).

Manipulative-based approaches, such as massage therapy,
have been studied with respect to chronic pain syndromes. These
modalities may offer some benefit—they have been shown to
reduce stress and improve mood. Physical therapy is no longer
considered to be an alternative approach and is an important part
of multidisciplinary therapy for chronic pelvic pain.

Mind–body-based medicine includes various "top down"
approaches, including hypnotherapy, meditation, and yoga. Mind–
body-based therapy, such as cognitive, behavioral, and relaxation
approaches, with or without biofeedback is now approaching
"mainstream" status and has been studied extensively for chronic
pain conditions but there are few RCTs. Hypnotherapy and cognitive behavioral therapy have been investigated and are useful in
the treatment of IBS, chronic pelvic pain, and vulvodynia. Meditation is safe, and may help reduce the stress and anxiety that are
often associated with chronic pain syndromes. Yoga has become
increasingly mainstream over the past decades and is thought to
improve overall well-being by increasing strength and stamina as
well as promoting self-awareness and stress reduction. A review
of seven RCTs that evaluated the efficacy of yoga in the treatment of chronic low back pain was published in 2011 (102). In
five of the seven trials, yoga was found to improve functionality,

although the effects on the reduction of pain symptoms are variable. Additional studies are necessary to determine a benefit of yoga for patients with chronic pelvic pain, but adverse effects are rare (103). There is some limited evidence suggesting that biofeedback may lead to improvement of dysmenorrhea, pelvic floor pain, and myofascial pain (101).

Acupuncture and transcutaneous electrical nerve stimulations (TENS) are among the most well studied modalities of CAM for chronic pelvic pain. A 2010 review of 27 studies demonstrated efficacy of acupuncture compared with pharmacologic therapy in the treatment of menstrual pain and also reported that adverse effects were rare (104). A meta-analysis of nine RCTs found that high-frequency TENS and also acupuncture were effective for the treatment of dysmenorrhea (105).

Although TENS in not currently recommended for the treatment of lower back pain or myofascial pain, small randomized trials suggest its utility in the treatment of dysmenorrhea as well as several neuropathic conditions, such as postherpetic neuralgia and vulvodynia (106).

Special Concerns for Older Women

Chronic pelvic pain in older women is not generally caused by reproductive system pathology. However, because of the increased risk of cancer that involves the reproductive, GI, and GU tracts, malignancy should be ruled out based on the patient's history, examination, and appropriate imaging or tissue biopsy results in this population. Neurologic, rheumatologic, and myofascial diagnoses are more prevalent. Chronic injuries, muscle atrophy and decreased mobility, polypharmacy, poor sleep, and cognitive impairment represent particular challenges for pain management in this age group.

In managing pain in older women, it is important to remain cognizant of the physiologic changes that occur in older patients. Alterations in pharmacokinetics are associated with aging. The decrease in lean body mass, increase in body fat, and decrease in albumin levels may significantly change the amount of active treatment agent available. Even more significant is a substantial reduction in the body's clearance capacity for most drugs, resulting from age-related decline in kidney function. Creatinine level alone is not an accurate marker of clearance particularly in older adults because normally creatinine levels decrease with age and with a decrease of lean muscle mass. Creatinine level should be calculated based on the Cockcroft–Gault formula (as follows) and the dose of medications that are cleared primarily by the kidney should be adjusted accordingly:

$$\text{Creatinine Clearance} = (140 - \text{Age}) \times \text{Mass (kg)}/\\ (72 \times \text{Serum Creatinine [mg/dL]})$$

The result is multiplied by 0.85 for female patients.

The physiologic changes in older patients also may alter their pharmacodynamic sensitivity. For example, NSAIDs in these patients must be used with caution, particularly in those with preexisting reduction in renal function because they may precipitate acute renal failure. These drugs also increase sodium retention and may interfere with generation of vasodilatory prostaglandins and may aggravate hypertension, thus they should be used with caution in women with preexisting hypertension. Gastrointestinal bleeding also is a concern. Another area of concern is opioids. Older adults may be more susceptible than the general population to the respiratory and CNS depression that can be caused by these agents (see Box 1).

Although older adults have been shown to respond well to antidepressants, particularly SSRIs, they are more susceptible to their adverse effects. This is particularly true for TCAs, in which anticholinergic effects typically are more severe. When TCAs are necessary, selection of an agent with less antimuscarinic effect, such as nortriptyline or desipramine, may be helpful.

Older patients often have numerous medical conditions, and may be prescribed a variety of medications sometimes from different physicians. It is important to document and maintain an accurate record of the patient's medications and supplements, both prescribed and those sold over-the-counter. The pharmacists and online databases can help avoid potentially toxic or dangerous drug interactions, especially for patients prescribed anticoagulants, antihypertensives, or centrally active drugs that affect balance and cognition. In a large meta-analysis of the effects of various medications on the risk of fall in patients older than 70 years, narcotics, antidepressants, and benzodiazepines were associated with an increased risk whereas NSAIDs were not found to increase the risk of fall.

Special Considerations for Medication Management

A wide range of medications has been used to manage acute and chronic pain. Analgesic therapy for pelvic pain starts with NSAIDs. Inhibition of prostaglandin synthesis ameliorates the pain of dysmenorrhea as well as pain associated with endometriosis and leiomyomas, and can be very effective when these pathologies are present. If stronger medication is needed, narcotics can be helpful.

Pain Medication Abuse and Addiction

Despite significant analgesic effects of narcotics, physicians often are reluctant to prescribe them to patients out of concerns for potential abuse. The continuum begins with the development of dependence and tolerance and continues to abuse and addiction.

Drug dependence of the opioid type is marked by a relatively specific withdrawal or abstinence syndrome. Just as there are pharmacologic differences between the various opioids, there are also differences in psychologic dependence and the severity of withdrawal effects. For example, withdrawal from dependence on a strong agonist is associated with more severe withdrawal signs and symptoms than withdrawal from a mild or moderate agonist.

Manifestations of tolerance typically appear approximately after 2–3 weeks of frequent exposure to the typical therapeutic doses. However, development of tolerance after the initial opioid dose also is possible. To delay the development of tolerance, an opioid should be combined with a nonopioid analgesic. Once a patient does develop tolerance, a different opioid or a drug holiday should be considered to prevent the development of addiction to a particular opioid while maintaining the effective pain control.

Several models have been proposed to explain addiction, including impairment of neurochemical or behavioral processes or genetic predisposition to certain behaviors. Addiction in the context of pain treatment with opioids is characterized by a persistent pattern of dysfunctional opioid use that may involve any or all of the following:

- Adverse consequences associated with the use of opioids
- Loss of control over the use of opioids (craving for an opioid, the need to use the opioid for effects other than pain relief, and preoccupation with obtaining more opioids despite adequate analgesia)
- Drug-seeking behavior (requesting medication from multiple health care providers or requests for early refill)

Addiction should not be confused with pseudoaddiction. This behavioral pattern is similar to opioid addiction (eg, a patient exhibits a compulsive interest in the use of opioids), but is caused by inadequate treatment of pain and resolves when pain is appropriately managed.

PREVENTION OF DRUG ADDICTION AND ABUSE

The risk of addiction has been low in patients with chronic pain. However, if this risk represents a significant problem, especially in the patients with a history of substance abuse, the opioid use may be avoided by prescribing a nonopioid drug that has worked for the patient in the past at a minimum effective dose and readjusting the dosage as needed thereafter. If an opioid must be prescribed to a patient with a known opioid addiction or long-term use is anticipated, a written contract should be signed between the patient and the physician or a clinic. The contract should include the following statements:

- The patient agrees to allow the clinic access to prior records.
- Only one physician should prescribe all narcotics and if possible only one pharmacy should dispense medications.
- No changes in drug dose are allowed without prior discussion with the physician.

- Early refills and replacements of the prescriptions are not allowed.
- The patient should abstain from use of alcohol and illegal drugs.
- The patient should consent to random urine and blood tests when asked. Tests may include screening for use of illegal substances.
- The patient is required to bring the unused medication to each clinic visit.
- The patient should agree to be evaluated by a psychologist or psychiatrist while taking opioids for pain, if requested.

ADEQUATE PAIN MANAGEMENT IN PATIENTS WITH A HISTORY OF DRUG ABUSE

The general pain management plan for patients with a history of substance abuse or for any patient given a narcotic for chronic pain includes the following actions (107):

- Pain management should be maximized with nonopioid and nonpharmacologic interventions, such as nerve block or neuraxial analgesia, TENS, and physical therapy.
- The patient's cognitive level, quality of life, willingness to cooperate, presence or absence of psychologic disorders, and history of prior drug treatment should be assessed.
- The patient may need assessment by a psychologist or to enter an addiction treatment program, preferably one experienced in the care of patients with pain.
- If all other options are exhausted, consideration of opioid management may be appropriate. Clear goals should be defined and agreed upon as outlined earlier in this section.

In selecting the best dose of opioid analgesic for patients with a history of substance abuse, if possible, a physician should start with the drug that has worked for the patient in the past and follow these steps:

1. The drug should be prescribed at a dose that seems appropriate for the condition causing pain.
2. The objective is to settle on a dose that provides adequate pain relief (it would not be possible to eliminate the pain totally) at the minimal dose possible.

3. Sometimes, pain could be controlled with the as-needed dose; otherwise, the patient should be prescribed a scheduled regimen.

4. If the patient requires too many doses for breakthrough pain, she may benefit from long-acting narcotics to provide a steady level of pain control. The risk of abuse is still present with the use of long-acting narcotics.

5. The need for breakthrough doses should be regularly assessed and the long-acting opioid dose adjusted.

6. Initially, the medication should be dispensed at a 1-week supply.

7. In unusual circumstances, such as trauma, the dose of narcotics should be adjusted accordingly.

Clinic visits initially should be weekly, and then monthly. Chart documentation is important for optimal patient care and for medical–legal reasons. Documentation includes the reason the patient is taking the drug; the prescribed dosage of the medication; its efficacy and adverse effects; patient's functional status; adherence to the contractual agreement; any drug seeking behaviors; and reason for change in drug or dosage.

Reproductive Concerns

The use of teratogens in the management of chronic pelvic pain in pregnancy must be avoided, especially in the first trimester. However, there are many situations in which the use of pharmacotherapy is appropriate and necessary. The effect of pregnancy on preexisting pain is largely dependent on its etiology.

PREGNANCY-RELATED PAIN AND CHRONIC PAIN MANAGEMENT IN PREGNANT WOMEN

Typical management strategies for pregnancy-related pain include an initial trial of acetaminophen. A short course of NSAIDs (less than 48 hours) is acceptable in the first and second trimesters, as is a limited course of narcotics. Patients with preexisting pain symptoms caused by an underlying condition, such as diabetes or a rheumatologic disease, or those who are already undergoing treatment for a chronic pain condition should be treated in conjunction with the internist or appropriate specialist.

Musculoskeletal pain, such as chronic back pain, often is exacerbated by the weight gain and increased joint laxity associated with pregnancy. Hormone-associated pain, such as dysmenorrhea or endometriosis, usually is improved during pregnancy in the absence of cyclic hormonal stimulus. Inflammatory pain processes, such as those attributed to underlying rheumatologic or autoimmune conditions, can improve or deteriorate during pregnancy.

The most common pain reported during pregnancy is back pain, present in approximately 50% of patients at some point in pregnancy, with the most frequently affected sites reported as low back area, sacroiliac area, or both (108). Accentuation of lumbar lordosis and physiologic relaxation of the ligaments of the pelvic joints to accommodate the gravid uterus are the main causes. Typical low back and pelvic pain of pregnancy begins at approximately 16–18 weeks of gestation. Reserach has failed to show an association between several factors, including parity, estimated fetal weight, maternal age, and maternal weight gain and the development of back pain during pregnancy.

In the absence of preterm contractions, evaluation includes a thorough history and physical examination, including back and neurologic examination. Exclusion of serious pathology in the pregnant patient commonly is the responsibility of the obstetrician–gynecologist. Risk factors associated with atypical and worrisome pain during pregnancy include a history of trauma, drug abuse, acquired immune deficiency disease, fever, and systemic or neurologic symptoms. Radicular symptoms are commonly present during pregnancy, with an incidence of 1 in 10,000, but studies have not shown increased lumbar disc herniations or abnormalities compared with nonpregnant women. It has been theorized that radiating pain may be due to pressure on the lumbosacral nerves by the fetus.

On physical examination, a straight leg raise that causes low back pain with or without radiation to the ipsilateral lower extremity suggests either sacroiliac subluxation or disc herniation. Unilateral absence of patellar reflex is consistent with lumbar nerve root compression. Neurologic findings in the evaluation of pain during pregnancy should prompt consultation with a neurologist.

Plain radiography contributes vital information, primarily when fracture, dislocation, and destructive lesions of the bone are suspected. Pregnancy is not an absolute contraindication to radiographic evaluation, and exposure to the fetus of less than 10 rads has not been associated with an increase in mental or growth abnormalities. Magnetic resonance imaging also may play a role in establishing a diagnosis in a pregnant patient with symptoms or signs suggestive of nerve involvement. Electromyography (EMG) and nerve conduction studies may be necessary in the setting of new onset low-back pain associated with sensory or motor symptoms. However, given the possibility of nerve involvement, the use of MRI and EMG should be decided in consultation with a neurologist.

Neuropathic pain usually is unaffected by pregnancy but pudendal neuropathy and lateral femoral cutaneous neuropathy, also known as meralgia paresthetica, can develop during pregnancy or after delivery. Meralgia paresthetica is a purely sensory neuropathy caused by compression of the lateral femoral cutaneous nerve under or within the inguinal ligament. It is relatively common, and is attributed to the increased abdominal girth and lumbar lordosis associated with pregnancy. Typical symptoms include tingling and numbness of the lateral thigh. Treatment is supportive, and spontaneous recovery postpartum is expected. However, if discomfort is persistent and bothersome, patients may be treated with amitriptyline or local anesthetic injection or patches at the inguinal ligament (109). Chronic GI and GU pain conditions often are unaffected by pregnancy with persistence of the prepregnancy pain patterns.

Pharmacologic Management. The most crucial period for minimizing maternal exposure to pharmacologic agents is from 4–10 weeks before conception through 10 weeks of gestation, during organogenesis. Nevertheless, often there are reservations on the part of both the clinician and the patient regarding the use of medication for pain control during pregnancy.

Nonsteroidal Antiinflammatory Drugs

Although aspirin has been the most studied NSAID during pregnancy, most of the NSAIDs, including indomethacin, ibuprofen, and naproxen, have not been associated with an increased risk of congenital defects. The concern with their consistent use during pregnancy, especially during the third trimester, is related to the risk of oligohydramnios and antepartum closure of the ductus arteriosus leading to pulmonary hypertension. Analgesic doses of aspirin (greater than 300 mg daily) should be used with caution because they may increase the risk of intracranial hemorrhage in neonates, particularly before 35 weeks of gestation. Ketorolac has not been sufficiently studied to support its use during pregnancy.

Opioids

Two large studies have examined the effects of narcotic use in pregnancy. The larger of the two studies, the Collaborative Perinatal Project, included more than 50,000 pregnancies with more than 500 cases of first-trimester exposure to various narcotics (110). Only codeine showed a statistically significant increase in the rate of malformations, particularly respiratory malformations. However, other opioids, such as ethadone, oxycodone, and hydroxycodone, were not associated with an increased teratogenic risk. The smaller study, the Michigan Medicaid Study, reported no teratogenic effects in 289 infants exposed to oxycodone in utero (111). With persistent use throughout the pregnancy, neonates may experience withdrawal symptoms, which are dose dependent. Morphine, codeine, meperidine, tramadol, hydrocodone, fentanyl, propoxyphene, and oxymorphone are all pregnancy category C drugs, and should be used with caution and only if their benefits are thought to outweigh their risks.

Antidepressants

Although antidepressants are commonly prescribed in pregnancy for the management of mood disorders, there is rarely an indication for use of antidepressants in pregnancy for the treatment of pain in women without a preexisting condition. As previously discussed, TCAs have been used for the treatment of neuropathic pain syndromes. Most of these agents (amitriptyline, nortriptyline, and imipramine) are pregnancy category D agents known to be teratogenic in animal studies and associated with case reports of neonatal limb deformities in humans. The SSRI paroxetine also belongs in pregnancy category D and has been associated with an increase in major malformations, particularly cardiac defects. Fluoxetine and most other SSRIs are pregnancy category C. The American Academy of Pediatrics considers antidepressants to have unknown risk during lactation. Fluoxetine and most other

SSRIs are pregnancy category C. Fluoxetine has been the most studied SSRI in pregnancy. One review asserted that based on data published before 2000, no associations with major malformations were found (112). Some subsequent studies have raised questions with respect to paroxetine and cardiac anomalies. Although several reviews have shown no significant increase in rates of major malformations with other SSRIs, the findings with paroxetine have reignited studies in this area (113, 114). In a study of 228 women exposed to fluoxetine in the first trimester compared with 254 controls, there was no significant increase in minor malformations (115). Retrospective studies have suggested a possible association between SSRI use during late pregnancy and persistent pulmonary hypertension in the newborn; however, this is yet to be confirmed in larger studies (116). In general, SSRI and SNRI antidepressants should be used with caution in pregnancy, particularly in the first trimester, and clinicians must weigh the risks and benefits of use of this type of medication.

Anticonvulsants
Gabapentin, an anticonvulsant used to treat some neuropathic pain syndromes, has been minimally studied during pregnancy. It is currently classified as a pregnancy category C agent.

Nonpharmacologic Management. Nonpharmacologic management of pain is particularly appealing during pregnancy, when many practitioners may be more reluctant to prescribe pharmacologic agents as first-line treatment. Patient counseling about appropriate expectations of normal sensations throughout pregnancy is helpful.

Exercise and Body Support
Exercise has been supported throughout pregnancy and may help maintain muscle tone and posture. Aquatic exercises may be particularly useful given their low impact nature. A wedge shaped pillow used to support the abdomen when a woman is lying on her side has been shown to be beneficial for 57 of 92 pregnant women who experienced back pain at night (117).

Transcutaneous Electrical Nerve Stimulation
Transcutaneous electrical nerve stimulation has shown promise in the treatment of certain localized pain disorders. Transcutaneous electrical nerve stimulation has not been widely examined during

pregnancy, but a few small studies suggest it may be safe in patients with back and sacroiliac pain (118).

Acupuncture

It has been established that acupuncture is efficacious in the management of chronic low back pain in the nonpregnant patient (108). Several small studies have been conducted to evaluate acupuncture for pregnancy-related low back and pelvic girdle pain with conflicting results. A 2008 review of three RCTs that involved acupuncture used for the treatment of pregnancy-related back and pelvic pain found a significant reduction in pain, significantly decreased use of pain medication, and a trend toward improvement in function (119). One of the major disadvantages of acupuncture use during pregnancy is the need for long-term treatment, usually requiring at least six sessions.

Nonobstetric Surgery. Two percent of pregnancies are complicated by nonobstetric surgical problems, and approximately 50,000 pregnant patients undergo nonobstetric operations in the United States each year. Common conditions that might require operation during pregnancy include appendicitis, cholecystitis, breast diseases, thyroid diseases, and trauma. Pregnancy causes physiologic changes that can alter the patient's response to analgesics. Furthermore, the fetus also should be considered when planning perioperative pain management.

The pregnant patient has both a decreased functional residual capacity and an increased minute ventilation and oxygen consumption, which increase susceptibility to hypoxia and acidosis during periods of apnea and hypoxia. Blood volume and cardiac output increase as pregnancy progresses. Inferior venacaval compression by the gravid uterus in the supine position increases susceptibility to hypotension. Placement of the patient in the left lateral decubitus position decompresses the vena cava and improves venous return to the heart. Venous engorgement decreases the size of the epidural space, thereby reducing the dosage of local anesthetic and opioids required. As pregnancy progresses, lower esophageal sphincter pressure decreases, increasing the risk of vomiting and aspiration with sedation.

Four major fetal problems must be considered in planning maternal perioperative analgesia: 1) fetal asphyxia, 2) preterm labor and delivery, 3) teratogenicity, and 4) adverse fetal physiologic effects of maternal drugs. Fetal asphyxia can be prevented by maximizing maternal oxygen delivery. Hypotension and hypoxia must be avoided. Preterm labor and delivery can be difficult to prevent and often are related to the underlying disease process. Preterm labor is more commonly associated with abdominal operations and trauma than with any other factors. Risk of preterm labor is lowest if the operation is performed during the second trimester of pregnancy. Teratogenic drugs should not be used unless absolutely essential for maternal salvage. However, none of the opioids are teratogenic.

As a general rule, NSAIDs should not be used in late pregnancy because of the risk of premature closure of the ductus arteriosis. An exception is the use of low-dose aspirin in patients with previous spontaneous abortions from placental abnormalities. Opioids are generally safe analgesics for acute pain when used in pregnant women, although they can cause neonatal respiratory depression when used near the time of delivery. Morphine is a good choice, because there is extensive experience with its use, and small doses can be titrated to achieve satisfactory analgesia and minimize respiratory depression, although there is a high incidence of nausea and vomiting. Hydromorphone is the other choice. For patients with mild to moderate pain, treatment with small doses of intravenous (IV) narcotics is reasonable (1–2 mg of IV morphine for 2–4 hours or 0.2 mg of IV hydromorphone every 2–4 hours). This method is labor intensive for the nursing staff and may not provide optimal analgesia to control the patient's pain. Patient-controlled analgesia is associated with superior analgesia per drug dose, less risk of maternal respiratory depression, less placental drug transfer, a lower incidence of nausea and vomiting, and improved patient satisfaction. Basal doses of narcotics are not used in pregnancy because of the increased risk of respiratory depression. Morphine is given as a starting dose of 1 mg bolus with a 10-minute lockout or hydromorphone 0.2 mg bolus every 10 minutes (120).

Obstetric Pain Management

Patient-controlled epidural analgesia is becoming an increasingly common analgesic technique during labor. A combination of a local anesthetic and a narcotic provides fast onset of action and prolonged analgesia. Low doses of both drugs can be used, limiting systemic local anesthetic toxicity and total narcotic dosage. Bupivacaine is an excellent choice of local anesthetic because it is long lasting and protein bound, which limits placental transfer. Fentanyl or hydromorphone are the preferred narcotics because they are associated with a lower risk of delayed respiratory depression compared with morphine. Routine postoperative monitoring of all pregnant patients receiving either IV bolus analgesia, patient-controlled anesthesia, or patient-controlled epidural analgesia includes the use of supplemental oxygen and pneumatic stockings, elevation of the head of the bed to prevent reflux, and hourly monitoring of vital signs, pulse oximetry, and fetal heart rate for the first 16 hours and then every 2–4 hours, if stable. Monitoring for uterine contractions also should be performed initially and continued for up to 7 days in high-risk patients.

The management of acute pain after cesarean delivery has evolved considerably over the past decade. The general approach to pain management after cesarean delivery is shifting away from traditional opioid-based therapy toward a "multimodal" or "balanced" approach. Multimodal pain therapy involves the use of a potent opioid regimen, such as patient-controlled analgesia or neuraxial opioids, in combination with other classes of analgesics and local anesthetics. Theoretically, such combination allows for additive or even synergistic effects in reducing pain while decreasing the adverse effects produced by each class of drug because smaller drug doses are required. Typical analgesic regimens include opioids; nonopioid analgesics, such as acetaminophen; and NSAIDs, with the variable addition of local anesthetic techniques.

Primary regimens consist of a potent opioid analgesic, such as neuraxial morphine, administered at the time of cesarean delivery or IV patient-controlled anesthesia started in the immediate perioperative period after a loading dose of the opioid. Primary analgesic regimens generally provide the bulk of pain relief for most women during the first postoperative day and often during part of the second postoperative day.

Secondary analgesic regimens are started in the immediate postoperative period to supplement the analgesia provided by neuraxial morphine. These regimens typically consist of oral analgesics (codeine or oxycodone and acetaminophen) that are given either on a scheduled basis or by a patient request. Nonsteroidal antiinflammatory drugs are administered on a regular basis and are started immediately after cesarean delivery. Supplemental pain relief also may include the use of local anesthetic wound infiltration or nerve blocks at the end of cesarean delivery.

In general, the drugs used as part of the secondary regimen are continued as the major form of pain relief on the second and third postoperative days. Breakthrough pain may require the use of additional parenteral opioids or adjustment of the dosage of patient-controlled anesthesia. When neuraxial opioids are used as the primary regimen, the administration of additional parenteral opioids should be monitored closely because of the potential added risk of respiratory depression.

Neuraxial Morphine. Neuraxial morphine is considered the standard treatment for pain after cesarean delivery, with significant reductions in pain scores on the first postoperative day compared with patient-controlled anesthesia or IM opioid injections. Neuraxial morphine mediates selective spinal analgesia by binding to opioid receptors in the substantia gelatinosa of the dorsal horn of the spinal cord near the site of injection. The levels of opioid required to produce supraspinal effects by this route are less than those that cause nausea. Preservative-free morphine could be used in the intrathecal space during spinal analgesia or in the epidural space during epidural analgesia. The doses and onset of action are shown in Table 13.

Intrathecal Analgesia. Preservative-free morphine, fentanyl, and local anesthetics can be administered in combination at the

Table 13. Morphine Routes and Onsets of Action

Route	Dose	Onset of Action	Duration of Action	Side Effects
Intrathecal	0.2 mg	15–30 minutes	8–24 hours	Nausea, vomiting, pruritus, and respiratory depression
Epidural	3 mg	15–30 minutes	6–24 hours	Nausea, vomiting, pruritus, and respiratory depression

time of spinal anesthesia for cesarean delivery. Bupivacaine, 0.75%, with dextrose, 8.25%, (1.2–1.8 mL) and preservative-free morphine (0.2 mg) with or without fentanyl (10 micrograms) are effective combinations. Authors of a prospective study of more than 850 patients undergoing elective cesarean delivery reported that the use of morphine (0.2 mg) provided effective analgesia for the duration of 14–24 hours (121). During the first 24 hours, doses greater than 0.2 mg produced more adverse effects without improving the quality of analgesia. Smaller studies that examined the efficacy of low doses of intrathecal morphine suggest that further reductions in the dose are possible to avoid adverse effects, but that patients may require supplemental analgesia in the postoperative period (122, 123).

Epidural Opioids. At cesarean delivery, epidural morphine is administered after delivery of the infant. A dose of 3 mg is considered the lowest effective dose of morphine with the least adverse effects. Fentanyl and sufentanil have all been used successfully for epidural pain relief, but have a shorter duration of action than morphine and need frequent, repeated administration. After a single dose, the analgesic effect ranges from 60 minutes to 120 minutes.

Morphine Sulfate Extended-Release Liposome Injection. Morphine sulfate extended-release liposome injection is a morphine sulfate formulation enclosed in microscopic lipid-based particles. The particles gradually erode, releasing morphine over a period of time. It is approved only in the form of epidural injection. The onset of action is approximately 3 hours and the duration of action is 48 hours. For postoperative pain control after cesarean delivery, the dose is 10 mg or 15 mg. The same monitoring used for preservative-free morphine applies to a morphine sulfate extended-release liposome injection, except for longer duration (48 hours). The injection is applied as a single shot so it could be used in patients with the need for postoperative anticoagulation because there would be no indwelling epidural catheter. However, this morphine sulfate formulation is approved only for epidural use and cannot be coadministered with local anesthetics. Some delayed respiratory depression also can occur.

Intravenous Patient-Controlled Analgesia. Patient-controlled analgesia has been used in the management of postoperative pain for more than a decade. This modality is preferred to IM opioid injections because it overcomes the problems of inappropriate drug dosage and delay in drug administration. It provides an improved way of assessing the need for postoperative analgesia because patients medicate themselves to an acceptable level of comfort and control adverse effects without being overmedicated. Its success relies on both the patient and nurse education, the availability of pumps, and vigilance in recognizing inadequate analgesia and adjusting the dosage accordingly. The choice of opioid is based on availability, patient and institutional preference, drug costs, pharmacokinetic considerations, and side-effect profiles. Morphine and hydromorphone have been shown to provide effective analgesia. Patient-controlled analgesia should be combined with a secondary regimen started immediately after cesarean delivery.

Nonsteroidal Antiinflammatory Drugs. In general, an NSAID is the best secondary regimen and, when not contraindicated, is administered by way of rectal suppository, followed with regular oral doses of an NSAID and regular doses of acetaminophen while the patient is awake. When the patient-controlled anesthesia is discontinued (usually on the second postoperative day), the NSAID and acetaminophen should be continued on a schedule with the addition of an oral opioid, such as oxycodone or codeine, for breakthrough pain.

Adjuvant Local Anesthetic Techniques. The use of local anesthetic techniques, including wound infiltration, rectus sheath, and ilioinguinal iliohypogastric nerve blocks, have met with variable success after cesarean delivery. The effectiveness of these measures, if present, is generally limited to pain relief on the first day after surgery; they need to be supplemented with opioids and NSAIDs. Another nerve block that can be used for lower abdominal procedures, such as cesarean delivery, is transversus abdominis plane block. The anterior abdominal wall (skin, muscles, and parietal peritoneum) is innervated by the anterior rami of T-7–L-1. Terminal branches of these somatic nerves course through the lateral abdominal wall within a plane between the internal oblique and transversus abdominis muscles, known as the transversus abdominis plane. Therefore, a bilateral injection of local anesthetic can potentially provide bilateral analgesia to the skin, muscles, and parietal peritoneum of the anterior abdominal wall from T-7 to L-1 (124).

Safety and Adverse Effects. The major adverse effects of neuraxial morphine include pruritus, nausea and vomiting, urinary retention, and respiratory depression. The incidence of pruritus varies widely from 0% to 100% and occurs with varying degrees of severity. This adverse effect likely is the result of the cephalad spread of opioid in the cerebrospinal fluid to the trigeminal nucleus, which is located superficially in the medulla. Pruritus is easily treated by administering small doses of IV or IM nalbuphine, 5 mg, every 4–6 hours.

The incidence of nausea and vomiting after neuraxial opioids is at least 30%, which is the same for women receiving parenteral opioids. Antiemetics, such as IV ondansetron, 4 mg, every 4–6 hours, can be used.

Urinary retention, although a noted problem after use of intrathecal or epidural opioids, is less of a concern in patients after cesarean delivery because these women usually have an indwelling urinary catheter in the immediate perioperative period.

Respiratory depression is the most feared adverse effect of neuraxial opioid administration, although the incidence requiring intervention is 1% (similar to that found after IV and IM opioid injections). Clinically important, early respiratory depression occurs within 2 hours and is associated with epidural administration of lipophilic drugs, such as sufentanil, and is likely related to systemic drug absorption. Delayed respiratory depression is associated with the use of neuraxial morphine, usually occurring from 6 hours to 12 hours after epidural or intrathecal morphine administration, yet it may occur for up to 24 hours. Simple hourly measurement of the respiratory rate and pulse oximetry for the first 18–24 hours by a trained nurse in a regular postpartum area is considered an adequate and safe method of monitoring respiration in these patients. In the unlikely event that respiratory depression does occur, titrated doses of naloxone should be administered and the patient should be carefully monitored. Naloxone should be kept at the bedside and postpartum nursing staff should be trained in its administration with a prespecified protocol. Those considered at risk of respiratory depression include women with marked obesity and those receiving parenteral narcotics, in addition to relatively large doses of neuraxial morphine. These patients should receive very close postoperative surveillance.

Breast Milk Transfer. Nonsteroidal antiinflammatory drugs, acetaminophen, and opioids are transferred to breast milk in varying degrees. This secretion is facilitated by several factors including high lipid solubility, low molecular weight, minimal protein binding, and nonionized state. The neonatal dose of most medications is 1–2% of the maternal dose (117). Breast milk usually is synthesized and secreted within the first hour after breastfeeding. The use of these drugs in breastfeeding women generally is compatible with breastfeeding. Rare cases of neonatal adverse effects have been reported.

Most NSAIDs, including ibuprofen, naproxen, and ketorolac, have demonstrated insignificant concentrations in breast milk and are approved for use in breastfeeding women by the American Academy of Pediatrics. Aspirin should be avoided in breastfeeding women because it is metabolized much more slowly by the neonate than other analgesics. Indomethacin has been associated with neonatal seizures and nephrotoxicity and also should be avoided in breastfeeding women. Narcotics are minimally detected in breast milk and are acceptable for use in these women.

The American Academy of Pediatrics considers antidepressants to have an unknown risk during lactation. Tricyclic antidepressants, including amitriptyline, nortriptyline, and desipramine, are all excreted into human milk with infant exposure estimated at 1% of the maternal dose. One review reported that amitriptyline, nortriptyline, desipramine, and sertraline were not found in appreciable quantities in breast milk. Fluoxetine is excreted in human milk with a milk to plasma ratio of 0.3 (117). Although gabapentin has not been extensively studied during lactation, other commonly used anticonvulsants are minimally secreted in breast milk and are acceptable for use in breastfeeding women.

Management of Perioperative Pain

Surgical pain is a result of either inflammation caused by tissue injury or direct nerve injury during surgery. The goal of postoperative pain control is aimed at both reducing local inflammatory mediators as well as blocking pain sensation at a central level. Adequate pain management will not only prevent needless suffering, but also will reduce the risk of adverse outcomes (thromboembolic or pulmonary complications and development of chronic pain), maintain the patient's functional ability as well as psychological well-being, enhance quality of life, shorten hospital stay, and reduce the costs. The goal is to provide continuous pain relief and reassess the adequacy of pain control.

Assessment of pain in an adult patient relies on patient's self-report (numerical scale), which varies among patients depending on their pain tolerance. Although the physiologic parameters, such as blood pressure and heart rate, could be used as an indicator of pain, it would be more useful in acute postoperative settings. Also, patients with a history of chronic pain and narcotic use may not be hypertensive or tachycardic. Therefore, the numerical scale may be used to assess if the new pain regimen has decreased the pain score or made no difference.

One of the concerns and fears for patients undergoing surgery is how well their pain would be controlled. The use of opioids for chronic moderate to severe pain is increasing. These patients use narcotics for chronic benign pain or malignancy-related pain; other patients have a history of substance abuse. At some point these patients need surgery. The factors that make the perioperative pain management challenging are tolerance, dependence, withdrawal, and adverse effects of the drugs being used. Another group of patients that presents a challenge in perioperative pain management (although not to the same extent as the previous group) are the patients with high level of anxiety.

Other factors to be considered in perioperative pain management are the type of surgery and underlying medical conditions, such as the following:

- History of narcotic use, drug abuse, and severe anxiety
- Type of surgery (simple versus extensive)

- Underlying medical condition (respiratory, cardiac, or renal disease)

Patients with a history of chronic obstructive pulmonary disease would benefit from interventional pain management, such as epidural analgesia, to decrease the postoperative narcotic requirement. In patients with renal insufficiency, the dose of medications needs to be adjusted.

Overall preoperative planning and preparation consist of

- patient and family education
- treatment to reduce preexisting pain and anxiety
- adjustment or continuation of pain medication (sudden cessation may provoke a withdrawal syndrome)

In the ambulatory setting, patients generally are healthier, the procedures they undergo are relatively minor, and the postoperative pain is mild to moderate. Patients are either discharged the same day or stay for a 23-hour observation period. It is best to use multimodal analgesia (to decrease the narcotic requirement), such as infiltration of the wound with local anesthetic, peripheral nerve block, if possible, and the use of NSAIDs (eg, ketorolac), if not contraindicated. Opioid-tolerant patients may need to stay overnight for better pain control. This option should be discussed with the patient before the surgery (Table 14).

Opioids

In the immediate postoperative period, IV narcotics are commonly used, such as morphine, hydromorphone, and fentanyl. For moderate postoperative pain, it is important to administer a loading dose followed by intermittent injection. The usual loading dose of morphine, 2 mg (approximately 0.1–0.3 mg/kg), or hydromorphone 0.2–0.6 mg (0.01–0.03 mg/kg), typically is used.

Intravenous opioid therapy often is administered as patient-controlled anesthesia through a pump, which offers many benefits, including ease of administration and decrease in medication errors. A 2006 review of 55 RCTs that compared patient-controlled anesthesia with standard IV injection of narcotics revealed significantly improved pain control and patient satisfaction in the patient-controlled anesthesia group without a difference in

Table 14. Perioperative Pain Management With Opioids

Setting of Surgery	Opioid-Naïve Patient	Opioid-Tolerant Patient
Ambulatory		
Same day discharge	Narcotic, eg, hydrocodone, in combination with acetaminophen	Multimodal analgesia; patient may need stronger or higher dose of narcotic; consider morphine or oxycodone
Overnight observation	Intravenous narcotic (patient-controlled analgesia or as needed); discharge with a prescription for narcotic, eg, hydrocodone, in combination with acetaminophen	Continue home pain medication or adjust the intravenous patient-controlled analgesia narcotic dose; discharge with stronger or higher dose of narcotic; consider morphine or oxycodone
Inpatient setting		
Minor procedure	Intravenous patient-controlled analgesia (by demand only)	Epidural analgesia (if patient is a candidate) or intravenous patient-controlled analgesia
Major procedure	Epidural analgesia (if patient is a candidate) or intravenous patient-controlled analgesia	Epidural analgesia (if patient is a candidate) or intravenous patient-controlled analgesia; patient may need rescue doses of parenteral opioids

adverse effects or length of hospital stay (125). Bolus injection doses can be titrated upwards, but continuous dosages should be avoided. Patients must be monitored for respiratory depression. Patient-controlled anesthesia or intermittent injection of fentanyl can be used as an alternative agent in patients with morphine allergy; however, the short half-life of this drug results in sub-optimal length of analgesia and limits its use. Intravenous opioids typically are discontinued once the patient is tolerating an oral diet, and there are several formulation options available. The choice of opioid for patient-controlled anesthesia is guided by the same principles as the choice of any other potent opioid, and the data are limited to indicate that one is preferred over another. If excessive adverse effects occur with one drug, a change to another drug might produce a better effect. In one study that compared hydromorphone, morphine, and fentanyl for acute postoperative pain management, the patients taking fentanyl reported lower rates of common opioid-induced adverse reactions than those in the other groups (126). When compared with the patients in the morphine group those in the hydromorphone group had lower pruritus and urinary retention although the difference was not statistically significant. Another study that compared morphine and hydromorphone showed similar side effect profiles for the two drugs, but slightly improved mood with hydromorphone (127). Another study found early euphoria followed by mood worsening with fentanyl compared with morphine. The requisite oral dose of narcotic agent may be estimated based on the 24-hour patient-controlled anesthesia.

Opioid regimens for patients in the postoperative period are given in Table 15. In opioid-tolerant patients, consider the following:

- Intravenous patient-controlled anesthesia should be initiated in the recovery room. Usually, in addition to demand boluses, the basal rate is needed. For demand boluses, a higher dose of narcotics should be administered and for basal rate, one fourth to one third of the patient's daily narcotic requirement is given.

- The use of a fentanyl patch should be either continued or an equianalgesic dose added to patient's pain regimen.

- Until the patient is able to tolerate oral intake, the daily narcotic dose should be converted to parenteral form, and she may require a 30–100% increase in the baseline dose (Table 13). Furthermore, a patient needs to be monitored closely when using high doses of narcotics or converting from oral to parenteral form. It is better to underestimate the conversion dose, reassess the patient frequently, and increase the dose as needed.

Table 15. Dose Regimen for Patient-Controlled Analgesia

Drug	Bolus Dose (mg)	Lock Out Time (Minutes)
Morphine	1–2	5–15
Hydromorphone	0.1–0.2	5–10
Fentanyl*	0.01–0.02	5–10

*Fentanyl is rarely used for intravenous patient-controlled analgesia because it is very potent. It should be considered only for patients with allergy to morphine and hydromorphone.

- If not contraindicated, ketorolac should be added to the patient's pain regimen. Ketorolac is a strong NSAID, without the narcotic adverse effects.

Nonsteroidal Antiinflammatory Drugs

Nonsteroidal antiinflammatory drugs have been shown to reduce the amount of opioids used in the postoperative period. A 2009 Cochrane review evaluated 72 studies in 66 reports that included 5,804 participants who took ibuprofen and 3,382 participants who took placebo (128). At 200 mg and 400 mg, respectively, 46% and 55% of patients experienced at least a 50% reduction in pain. This result is comparable with that of other analgesics commonly used for postoperative pain. Limited data for ibuprofen used in doses of 600 mg and 800 mg were compatible with this trend. This review demonstrated a nonsignificant trend for fewer participants to need rescue medication within 6 hours. Both of these results indicate that the higher doses give more prolonged pain relief than lower doses (128).

Ketorolac is an intravenously or intramuscularly administered NSAID with potent analgesic effects. Intramuscular ketorolac, 30 mg, produces analgesia that is equivalent to 10 mg of morphine or 100 mg of meperidine. An important benefit of ketorolac-induced analgesia is the absence of respiratory or CV depression. However, ketorolac should not be used for more than 5 days. During the postoperative period, the lowest effective dose for the shortest duration should be used. Ketorolac is contraindicated in the postoperative period in patients with an increased risk of bleeding because ketorolac affects platelet aggregation and hemostasis. It also should be used with caution in patients with history of peptic ulcer, elderly patients, and hypovolemic patients because of the risk of renal toxicity.

Regional Anesthesia

Neuraxial anesthesia offers unique benefits in the intraoperative and postoperative setting. When used intraoperatively, both epidural as well as spinal anesthesia have been shown to reduce the use of IV narcotics in the immediate postoperative period. Neuraxial anesthesia is thought to function by suppressing neuropeptide secretion from within the spinal cord. Spinal or intrathecal anesthesia can be used in a single injection to provide intra-operative anesthesia, and in sufficient dosages, it may provide adequate pain control for up to 24 hours. Postoperative epidural anesthesia may be particularly useful for extensive surgery or in a patient with a history of chronic opioid dependence.

Local Anesthesia

Preoperative injection of a local anesthetic has been shown to decrease incision-site pain around small laparoscopy incisions, but not around laparotomy sites. One pilot case–control study showed that intraperitoneal irrigation with bupivacaine (long-acting local anesthetic) significantly reduced postoperative IV analgesic requirements after laparoscopy compared with control (0.5 mg versus 7.17 mg) without differences in pain scores or length of hospital stay (129). Continuous wound perfusion using the ON-Q system also has been evaluated as a form of local anesthesia. A double-blinded placebo controlled trial compared 72-hour continuous wound perfusion through the ON-Q pain management system of the local anesthetic 0.5% bupivacaine (study group) or 0.9% sodium chloride (control group) (130). There was no difference in overall postoperative pain scores. Patients in the study group required less narcotic than those in the control group. However, there was no significant difference in length of hospitalization or time to first bowel movement.

Overdose in the Perioperative Period

Several of the medications used in pain control are susceptible to overuse, even to the point of toxicity. It is important to recognize the signs of a possible overdose involved in medications prescribed. Patients with overdose may present with altered mental status, coma, or arrest. Initial management involves stabilization of the patient with possible endotracheal intubation. Serial vital sign measurements should be obtained. If possible, a list of medications, any intake, including food, and medical history should be reviewed, either directly with the patient or with the patient's relatives. Several laboratory tests may be ordered to help elucidate the causative agent if identification by history is not possible. These include measurements of electrolytes and arterial blood gas and electrocardiography. The patient care should be managed in the critical care setting in conjunction with an intensive care physician.

Discharge Plan

Discharge medications should be planned as soon as possible, especially in opioid-tolerant patients, so the discharge will not be delayed. As soon as the patient is able to tolerate oral intake, an oral pain regimen should be administered. In narcotic-naïve patients, parenteral medication can be discontinued and oral nonopioid or opioid analgesics started. In opioid-tolerant patients some overlap time should be allowed between tapering down the parenteral opioids and starting oral opioids. Generally, in these patients, the usual home oral pain regimen needs to be restarted and supplemented with extra doses of opioids for postoperative pain control.

The prescribing physician should discuss the following with patients who are being discharged with a prescription for narcotic medications:

- Activities requiring mental alertness or coordination should be avoided until the drug effects are realized.
- The next dose of narcotic should be avoided if somnolence or signs or symptoms of respiratory depression occur.
- The drug should not be discontinued suddenly. The patient can decrease the dose by 25–50% every 2 days if the pain decreases.
- The use of concomitant CNS depressants and alcohol should be avoided.

A patient also should be advised not to take any other acetaminophen during treatment if using combinations of narcotics and acetaminophen.

Management of Terminal and End-of-Life Pain

Effective pain management in the terminally ill patient requires an understanding of pain control strategies. Adequate pain management improves the ability to cope with therapy and improves nutrition and sleep (131). The goal is to maintain or improve the quality of daily life. Ongoing assessment of pain is crucial and it also is important to determine the following aspects:

- If the pain is acute or chronic and nociceptive or neuropathic
- Which other pain medications the patient has used and what are their adverse effects
- If the patient is able to tolerate an oral regimen or not

Depending on the severity and the type of pain, the regimen may consist of nonopioids (NSAIDs), opioids, and adjuvants. Generally, patients with cancer pain have a combination of baseline pain and breakthrough pain (Table 16). For the baseline

Table 16. Opioid Analgesics for Baseline Pain and Breakthrough Pain Management

Patient Characteristics	Baseline Pain (Scheduled)	Breakthrough Pain (As Needed)
Patient able to take oral medication	Methadone Morphine sulfate controlled release Oxycodone hydrochloride Morphine sulfate	Morphine sulfate Oxycodone Hydrocodone
Patients not able to tolerate oral intake	Intravenous route—basal rate on intravenous patient-controlled analgesia (hydromorphone hydrochloride or morphine) Enteral route (through G or J tube)—methadone (crushed); morphine sulfate extended release capsules (capsule or beads should not be chewed, crushed, or dissolved): • Kadian—the capsule may be opened and contents sprinkled on a small amount of applesauce or administered through a 16 French gastrostomy tube • Avinza—the capsule may be opened and bead contents sprinkled on small amount of applesauce Transdermal route—fentanyl patch	Intravenous route—demand dose administered through intravenous patient-controlled analgesia hydromorphone (hydrochloride or morphine) Enteral route—elixir or crushed: morphine sulfate, oxycodone, or hydrocodone Submucosal route—fentanyl lollipops, lozenges, or tablets

pain, a pain regimen that allows the delivery of the drug around the clock should be considered. For the breakthrough pain, the pain medication should have a rapid onset and short duration and be used as needed so it would match the peaks of time of the day when the patient has breakthrough pain. If a significant amount of medication for breakthrough pain is already being administered, the baseline dose of extended-release analgesic medication should be increased. The goal is to prevent analgesic gaps and to allow the patient to take the medication less frequently. Patients able to take medications orally should be prescribed the extended-release analgesic that can be taken every 12 hours or once a day. Such analgesic provides prolonged and consistent plasma concentration, which results in better night-time pain control and less clock watching and is more convenient for the patient (Table 17). When changing the narcotics or the route of administration, it is safer to use a lower dose than an equianalgesic dose. Also, during this period the patient should be monitored and reassessed more frequently.

A psychiatrist should be involved in the care of terminally ill patients with chronic pain because many of these patients may experience anxiety or depression. Patients with chronic pain are more likely to report depressive symptoms, and their depression may be more severe and resistant to treatment than in other patients. Pain, depression, and pain-related depression increase disability in physical illness, amplify pain and other symptoms,

Table 17. Opioid Analgesics

Drug	Route	Starting Dose	Interval	Comments
Fentanyl lollipops and lozenges	Transmucosal	200 micrograms (may repeat only one more dose in 30 minutes)	4 hours (maximum dose, less than four units per day)	Should not be used in the management of acute or postoperative pain, should be used only in the management of breakthrough pain; in cancer patients with opioid tolerance, the dose can be escalated to reach analgesic effect, and should not be chewed

(continued)

Table 17. Opioid Analgesics *(continued)*

Drug	Route	Starting Dose	Interval	Comments
Fentanyl buccal tablet	Transmucosal	100 micrograms (may repeat only one more dose in 30 minutes)	4 hours (maximum dose, less than four units per day)	Higher bioavailability than lozenges (100-microgram tablet equals 200-microgram lozenge), should not be used in the management of acute or postoperative pain, should be used only in the management of breakthrough pain; in cancer patients with opioid tolerance, the dose can be escalated to reach analgesic effect, and should not be chewed
Fentanyl	Transdermal	12.5 micrograms per hour (the dose of 25 micrograms per hour is roughly equivalent to 45–134 milligrams per 24 hours of oral morphine)	72 hours	Should be used only in the management of moderate to severe chronic pain in opioid-tolerant patients requiring continuous opioid therapy; 12 hours onset and offset delay
Morphine sulfate (Avinza)	Oral	30 mg (in opioid-naïve patients, increments should not exceed 30 mg every 4 days)	24 hours	Contains both immediate-release and extended-release agents
Morphine sulfate extended release (Kadian)	Oral	20 mg (in opioid-naïve patients, increments should not exceed 20 mg every other day)	12–24 hours	

and shorten life expectancy. Like depression, anxiety has a complex relationship with pain, and they both have deleterious effects on sleep, coping, and expectations of pain relief. Given the frailty of these patients, SSRIs probably are a first choice for pharmacologic management of depression and anxiety, although nausea can be a side effect of SSRIs. However, nausea already is a common symptom in terminally ill patients. Another useful antidepressant is mirtazapine, which has an appetite stimulant action and sedative effects, making it popular with agitated patients and those who have lost considerable amounts of weight. Antidepressants are effective for many anxiety disorders and often have advantages over benzodiazepines, which are commonly used in palliative care. Psychostimulants have been suggested for use because of their quick onset of action (131). Although some evidence suggests that they are effective in treating depression, there is insufficient evidence to support their routine use for the treatment of depression in palliative care populations. Psychologic approaches need to be tailored to the patient's presenting difficulties and include behavioral activation, sleep hygiene, supportive psychotherapy, and family or marital techniques (132).

Conclusions

Pain is a complex symptom with many emotional overtones. Acutely, for example in the emergency room or during the perioperative period, pain generally is controlled effectively with judicious use of opioids, NSAIDs, and local anesthetics. However, when pain becomes a chronic condition, the biopsychosocial model should guide diagnosis and management. Peripheral and central neuroplastic changes maintain the chronic pain state. They are influenced by the individual patient's unique biochemistry, neuroanatomy, thoughts, emotions, and environment. This complicated, multisided disease requires multimodal, multidisciplinary treatment. The various visceral, somatic, and neurologic "pain generators" have to be identified and treated or down-regulated. Pharmacologic, surgical, cognitive–behavioral, relaxation, physical, and rehabilitation therapies and some complementary and alternative therapies are recommended and have been shown to be effective. Goals of therapy include reducing pain intensity and improving coping skills, mood, and overall quality of life.

Future Directions in Research and Therapy

Future research directions include identification of polymorphisms in genes coding for chemicals important in the modulation of inflammation and neural signaling (eg, neuropeptides, neurotransmitters, and inflammatory mediators) that can predispose an individual to develop chronic pain. This gene fingerprint could help tailor treatment and counsel patients about their risks. Discovery of gene polymorphisms for mediators, such as neurotransmitters and neuropeptides, involved in the control of mood and the stress response, in the inflammatory response, and in pain regulatory systems may allow for discovery of physiologic and psychologic risk factors, prevention, and treatments of chronic unexplained pain. Knowledge about the specific central processes underlying peripheral and central sensitization will lead to novel and more targeted pharmacologic approaches for pain alleviation. Further examination and understanding of these mechanisms will play a key role in the development of new treatment modalities for chronic pain. Currently, extensive research is underway to study a variety of chemokines (cytokines involved in chemotaxis), which also may contribute to chronic pain mechanisms, and may be useful targets. In addition to commonly used medications, the development of drugs that target other signaling pathways involved in neuropathic pain is crucial. For women with endometriosis and other estrogen mediated pain conditions, promising new SERMs may soon be available. Large, multicenter RCTs for various surgical procedures performed to treat chronic pelvic pain also are key.

Resources

American College of Obstetricians and Gynecologists' Patient Education
    Pamphlets

    Chronic Pelvic Pain (AP099)

    Dysmenorrhea (AP046)

    Endometriosis (AP013)

    Pelvic Inflammatory Disease (AP077)

    Premenstrual Syndrome (AP057)

    Vulvodynia (AP127)

    When Sex Is Painful (AP020)

Agencies and Organizations

    American Pain Society
    4700 W. Lake Ave.
    Glenview, IL 60025
    www.ampainsoc.org

    American Academy of Pain Management
    13947 Mono Way - #A
    Sonora, CA 95370
    www.aapainmanage.org

    International Pelvic Pain Society
    Two Woodfield Lake
    1100 E. Woodfield Rd. - Suite 520
    Schaumburg, IL 60173
    www.pelvicpain.org

    International Association for the Study of Pain
    111 Queen Anne Ave. N. - Suite 501
    Seattle, WA 98109-4955
    www.iasp-pain.org

    National Vulvodynia Association
    P.O. Box 4491
    Silver Spring, MD 20914-4491
    www.nva.org

Test Your Clinical Skills

Complete the answer sheet at the back of this book and return it to the American College of Obstetricians and Gynecologists to receive Continuing Medical Education credits. The answers appear on page 141.

Directions: Select the one best answer or completion.

1. Chronic pelvic pain is defined as existing for greater than how many months?
    A. 2
    B. 6
    C. 9
    D. 12

2. The distal fallopian tubes and upper ureters have common innervation with the
    A. upper bladder
    B. transverse colon
    C. ovary
    D. ascending colon

3. When normally innocuous stimuli result in pain, the condition is called
    A. allodynia
    B. hyperalgesia
    C. nociception
    D. neural plasticity

4. Irritation in one pelvic organ that decreases the threshold for sensation in a nearby structure due to inflammation is an example of
    A. crosstalk
    B. cross sensitization
    C. recruitment
    D. hyperalgesia

5. When taking Carnett's test results in diminished pain, it suggests that the origin of the pain is
   A. myofascial
   B. neuropathic
   C. psychogenic
   D. visceral

6. Which of the following has not been shown to relieve dysmenorrhea?
   A. Acupuncture
   B. Depot progestin
   C. Herbal therapy
   D. TENS

7. In an RCT of laser ablation for minimal and moderate endometriosis, what percentage of women reported improvement of pain at 1 year?
   A. 30
   B. 50
   C. 87
   D. 90

8. In the retrospective laparoscopic study of adhesions in patients with chronic pelvic pain compared with asymptomatic patients with infertility, the patients in the chronic pelvic pain group had
   A. more adhesions
   B. similar location and density of adhesions
   C. more dense adhesions
   D. more cul-de-sac adhesions

9. Which of the following symptoms is required to diagnose IBS using the Rome III criteria?
   A. Pain lasting 6 months
   B. Pain present for at least 3 days per month
   C. Pain relieved by defecation
   D. Presence of mucorrhea

10. The FDA-approved treament for IC/BPS is
    A. intravesical pentosan polysulfate sodium
    B. intravesical dimethylsulfoxide
    C. cyclosporine
    D. sacral neuromodulation

11. Which of the following signs or symptoms is least often found in patients with fibromyalgia?
    A. Fatigue
    B. Abnormal sleep pattern
    C. Joint inflammation
    D. Shoulder pain

12. Persistent sexual arousal disorder is associated with withdrawal from
    A. alprazolam
    B. amitriptyline
    C. trazodone
    D. gabapentin

13. Meralgia paresthetica results from compression of the nerve at
    A. inguinal ligament
    B. nerve root
    C. sacroiliac joint
    D. lumbosacral plexus

14. A study of more than 500 cases of first-trimester exposure to narcotics showed an increased incidence of malformations in patients receiving
    A. codeine
    B. hydroxycodone
    C. methadone
    D. oxycodone

15. According to the authors, which of the following antidepressants has the lowest association with fetal abnormalities when prescribed during pregnancy?
    A. Amitriptyline
    B. Fluoxetine
    C. Imipramine
    D. Paroxetin

16. An example of an opioid agonist is
    A. dihydrocodeine
    B. hydrocodone
    C. hydromorphone
    D. all of the above

17. Tolerance of opioids usually appears after what time period
    of frequent exposure?
    A. 3 days
    B. 3 weeks
    C. 6 weeks
    D. 2 months

18. For patients with a history of substance abuse, the authors
    recommend initial prescription of narcotics to last how long?
    A. 5 days
    B. 7 days
    C. 10 days
    D. 14 days

19. Ketorolac therapy for postoperative pain should be limited to
    how many days?
    A. 2
    B. 3
    C. 5
    D. 7

20. The authors recommend which of the following for treat-
    ment of pruritus associated with neuraxial morphine?
    A. Diphenhydramine
    B. Ibuprofen
    C. Nalbuphine
    D. Prednisone

References

1. Mathias SD, Kuppermann M, Liberman RF, Lipschutz RC, Steege JF. Chronic pelvic pain: prevalence, health-related quality of life, and economic correlates. Obstet Gynecol 1996;87:321–7. (Level III)

2. Latthe P, Latthe M, Say L, Gulmezoglu M, Khan KS. WHO systematic review of prevalence of chronic pelvic pain: a neglected reproductive health morbidity. BMC Public Health 2006;6:177. (Meta-analysis)

3. Howard FM. Chronic pelvic pain. Obstet Gynecol 2003;101:594–611. (Level III)

4. Zondervan KT, Yudkin PL, Vessey MP, Jenkinson CP, Dawes MG, Barlow DH, et al. The community prevalence of chronic pelvic pain in women and associated illness behaviour. Br J Gen Pract 2001;51:541–7. (Level II-3)

5. Latremoliere A, Woolf CJ. Central sensitization: a generator of pain hypersensitivity by central neural plasticity. J Pain 2009;10:895–926. (Level III)

6. Winnard KP, Dmitrieva N, Berkley KJ. Cross-organ interactions between reproductive, gastrointestinal, and urinary tracts: modulation by estrous stage and involvement of the hypogastric nerve. Am J Physiol Regul Integr Comp Physiol 2006;291:R1592–601. (Animal study)

7. Borsook D, Sava S, Becerra L. The pain imaging revolution: advancing pain into the 21st century. Neuroscientist 2010;16:171–85. (Level III)

8. Malykhina AP. Neural mechanisms of pelvic organ cross-sensitization. Neuroscience 2007;149:660–72. (Level III)

9. DeLeo JA, Tanga FY, Tawfik VL. Neuroimmune activation and neuroinflammation in chronic pain and opioid tolerance/hyperalgesia. Neuroscientist 2004;10:40–52. (Level III)

10. Eisenberg E, McNicol ED, Carr DB. Efficacy and safety of opioid agonists in the treatment of neuropathic pain of nonmalignant origin: systematic review and meta-analysis of randomized controlled trials. JAMA 2005;293:3043–52. (Meta-analysis)

11. Watson CP, Babul N. Efficacy of oxycodone in neuropathic pain: a randomized trial in postherpetic neuralgia. Neurology 1998;50:1837–41. (Level II-3)

12. Harati Y, Gooch C, Swenson M, Edelman S, Greene D, Raskin P, at al. Double-blind randomized trial of tramadol for the treatment of the pain of diabetic neuropathy. Neurology 1998;50:1842–6. (Level I)

13. Freeman R, Raskin P, Hewitt DJ, Vorsanger GJ, Jordan DM, Xiang J, et al. Randomized study of tramadol/acetaminophen versus placebo in painful diabetic peripheral neuropathy. CAPSS-237 Study Group. Curr Med Res Opin 2007;23:147–61. (Level I)

14. Gallagher RM. Management of neuropathic pain: translating mechanistic advances and evidence-based research into clinical practice. Clin J Pain 2006;22:S2–8. (Level III)

15. Jann MW, Slade JH. Antidepressant agents for the treatment of chronic pain and depression. Pharmacotherapy 2007;27:1571–87. (Level III)

16. Mays TA. Antidepressants in the management of cancer pain. Curr Pain Headache Rep 2001;5:227–36. (Level III)

17. Brown CS, Franks AS, Wan J, Ling FW. Citalopram in the treatment of women with chronic pelvic pain: an open-label trial. J Reprod Med 2008;53:191–5. (Level II-3)

18. Attal N, Brasseur L, Chauvin M, Bouhassira D. Effects of single and repeated applications of a eutectic mixture of local anaesthetics (EMLA) cream on spontaneous and evoked pain in post-herpetic neuralgia. Pain 1999; 81:203–9. (Level III)

19. Filler A. Diagnosis and management of pudendal nerve entrapment syndromes: impact of MR neurography and open MR-guided injections. Neurosurg Q 2008;18:1–6. (Level III)

20. Bremner JD, Bolus R, Mayer EA. Psychometric properties of the Early Trauma Inventory-Self Report. J Nerv Ment Dis 2007;195:211–8. (Level II-3)

21. Diatchenko L, Nackley AG, Slade GD, Fillingim RB, Maixner W. Idiopathic pain disorders--pathways of vulnerability. Pain 2006;123:226–30. (Level III)

22. Marjoribanks J, Proctor M, Farquhar C, Derks Roos S. Nonsteroidal anti-inflammatory drugs for primary dysmenorrhoea. Cochrane Database of Systematic Reviews 2010, Issue 1. Art. No.: CD001751. DOI: 10.1002/14651858.CD001751.pub2; 10.1002/14651858.CD001751.pub2. (Meta-analysis)

23. Wong Chooi L, Farquhar C, Roberts H, Proctor M. Oral contraceptive pill for primary dysmenorrhea. Cochrane Database of Systematic Reviews 2009, Issue 4. Art. No.: CD002120. DOI: 10.1002/14651858.CD002120.pub3; 10.1002/14651858.CD002120.pub3. (Meta-analysis)

24. Sulak PJ, Carl J, Gopalakrishnan I, Coffee A, Kuehl TJ. Outcomes of extended oral contraceptive regimens with a shortened hormone-free interval to manage breakthrough bleeding. Contraception 2004;70:281–7. (Level III)

25. Buck Louis GM, Hediger ML, Peterson CM, Croughan M, Sundaram R, Stanford J, et al. Incidence of endometriosis by study population and diagnostic method: the ENDO study. The ENDO Study Working Group. Fertil Steril 2011;96:360–5. (Level II-3)

26. Giudice LC, Kao LC. Endometriosis. Lancet 2004;364:1789–99. (Level III)

27. Al-Jefout M, Andreadis N, Tokushige N, Markham R, Fraser I. A pilot study to evaluate the relative efficacy of endometrial biopsy and full curettage in making a diagnosis of endometriosis by the detection of endometrial nerve fibers. Am J Obstet Gynecol 2007;197:578.e1–578.e4. (Level III)

28. Cornillie FJ, Oosterlynck D, Lauweryns JM, Koninckx PR. Deeply infiltrating pelvic endometriosis: histology and clinical significance. Fertil Steril 1990;53: 978–83. (Level III)

29. Allen C, Hopewell S, Prentice A. Nonsteroidal anti-inflammatory drugs for pain in women with endometriosis. Cochrane Database of Systematic Reviews 2009, Issue 2. Art.No.: CD004753. DOI: 10.1002/14651858. CD004753.pub3; 10.1002/14651858.CD004753.pub3. (Meta-analysis)

30. Hughes E, Brown J, Collins John J, Farquhar C, Fedorkow Donna M, Vanderkerchove P. Ovulation suppression for endometriosis for women with subfertility. Cochrane Database of Systematic Reviews 2007, Issue 3. Art. No.: CD000155. DOI: 10.1002/14651858.CD000155.pub2; 10.1002/14651858.CD000155.pub2. (Meta-analysis)

31. Vercellini P, Fedele L, Pietropaolo G, Frontino G, Somigliana E, Crosignani PG. Progestogens for endometriosis: forward to the past. Hum Reprod Update 2003;9:387–96. (Level III)

32. Somigliana E, Vigano P, Barbara G, Vercellini P. Treatment of endometriosis-related pain: options and outcomes. Front Biosci (Elite Ed) 2009;1:455–65. (Level III)

33. Hornstein MD, Surrey ES, Weisberg GW, Casino LA. Leuprolide acetate depot and hormonal add-back in endometriosis: a 12-month study. Lupron Add-Back Study Group. Obstet Gynecol 1998;91:16–24. (Level I)

34. Petta CA, Ferriani RA, Abrao MS, Hassan D, Rosa E Silva JC, Podgaec S, et al. Randomized clinical trial of a levonorgestrel-releasing intrauterine system and a depot GnRH analogue for the treatment of chronic pelvic pain in women with endometriosis. Hum Reprod 2005;20:1993–8. (Level I)

35. Nawathe A, Patwardhan S, Yates D, Harrison GR, Khan KS. Systematic review of the effects of aromatase inhibitors on pain associated with endometriosis [published arratum appears in BJOG 2008;115:1069]. BJOG 2008;115:818–22. (Level III)

36. Ferrero S, Camerini G, Seracchioli R, Ragni N, Venturini PL, Remorgida V. Letrozole combined with norethisterone acetate compared with norethisterone acetate alone in the treatment of pain symptoms caused by endometriosis. Hum Reprod 2009;24:3033–41. (Level II-3)

37. Kettel LM, Murphy AA, Morales AJ, Yen SS. Preliminary report on the treatment of endometriosis with low-dose mifepristone (RU 486). Am J Obstet Gynecol 1998;178:1151–6. (Level III)

38. Panay N. Advances in the medical management of endometriosis. BJOG 2008;115:814–7. (Level III)

39. Nasu K, Yuge A, Tsuno A, Narahara H. Simvastatin inhibits the proliferation and the contractility of human endometriotic stromal cells: a promising agent for the treatment of endometriosis. Fertil Steril 2009;92:2097–9. (Level III)

40. Vercellini P, Barbara G, Abbiati A, Somigliana E, Vigano P, Fedele L. Repetitive surgery for recurrent symptomatic endometriosis: what to do? Eur J Obstet Gynecol Reprod Biol 2009;146:15–21. (Level III)

41. Vercellini P, Crosignani PG, Somigliana E, Berlanda N, Barbara G, Fedele L. Medical treatment for rectovaginal endometriosis: what is the evidence? Hum Reprod 2009;24:2504–14. (Level III)

42. Hurd WW. Criteria that indicate endometriosis is the cause of chronic pelvic pain. Obstet Gynecol 1998;92:1029–32. (Level III)

43. Surrey ES, Hornstein MD. Prolonged GnRH agonist and add-back therapy for symptomatic endometriosis: long-term follow-up. Obstet Gynecol 2002; 99:709–19. (Level II-2)

44. Guzick DS, Huang LS, Broadman BA, Nealon M, Hornstein MD. Randomized trial of leuprolide versus continuous oral contraceptives in the treatment of endometriosis-associated pelvic pain. Fertil Steril 2011;95:1568–73. (Level I)

45. Kim HS, Malhotra AD, Rowe PC, Lee JM, Venbrux AC. Embolotherapy for pelvic congestion syndrome: long-term results. J Vasc Interv Radiol 2006;17:289–97. (Level II-3)

46. Beard RW, Kennedy RG, Gangar KF, Stones RW, Rogers V, Reginald PW, et al. Bilateral oophorectomy and hysterectomy in the treatment of intractable pelvic pain associated with pelvic congestion. Br J Obstet Gynaecol 1991;98: 988–92. (Level III)

47. Rapkin AJ. Adhesions and pelvic pain: a retrospective study. Obstet Gynecol 1986;68:13–5. (Level II-3)

48. Almeida OD Jr, Val-Gallas JM. Conscious pain mapping. J Am Assoc Gynecol Laparosc 1997;4:587–90. (Level III)

49. Swank DJ, Swank-Bordewijk SC, Hop WC, van Erp WF, Janssen IM, Bonjer HJ, et al. Laparoscopic adhesiolysis in patients with chronic abdominal pain: a blinded randomised controlled multi-centre trial. Lancet 2003;361:1247–51. (Level I)

50. Roman H, Hulsey TF, Marpeau L, Hulsey TC. Why laparoscopic adhesiolysis should not be the victim of a single randomized clinical trial. Am J Obstet Gynecol 2009;200:136.e1–136.e4. (Level III)

51. Olsen AL, Smith VJ, Bergstrom JO, Colling JC, Clark AL. Epidemiology of surgically managed pelvic organ prolapse and urinary incontinence. Obstet Gynecol 1997;89:501–6. (Level II-3)

52. Hanno P, Nordling J, Fall M. Bladder pain syndrome. Med Clin North Am 2011;95:55–73. (Level III)

53. Jones CA, Nyberg L. Epidemiology of interstitial cystitis. Urology 1997;49:2–9. (Level III)

54. Kim SH, Kim TB, Kim SW, Oh SJ. Urodynamic findings of the painful bladder syndrome/interstitial cystitis: a comparison with idiopathic overactive bladder. J Urol 2009;181:2550–4. (Level II-3)

55. Parsons CL. The potassium sensitivity test: a new gold standard for diagnosing and understanding the pathophysiology of interstitial cystitis. J Urol 2009;182:432–4. (Level III)

56. Hanno PM, Burks DA, Clemens JQ, Dmochowski RR, Erickson D, Fitzgerald MP, et al. AUA guideline for the diagnosis and treatment of interstitial cystitis/

bladder pain syndrome. Interstitial Cystitis Guidelines Panel of the American Urological Association Education and Research, Inc. J Urol 2011;185:2162–70. (Level III)

57. Chancellor MB, Yoshimura N. Treatment of interstitial cystitis. Urology 2004;63:85–92. (Level III)

58. Welk BK, Teichman JM. Dyspareunia response in patients with interstitial cystitis treated with intravesical lidocaine, bicarbonate, and heparin. Urology 2008;71:67–70. (Level III)

59. Perez-Marrero R, Emerson LE, Feltis JT. A controlled study of dimethyl sulfoxide in interstitial cystitis. J Urol 1988;140:36–9. (Level II-3)

60. Peeker R, Haghsheno MA, Holmang S, Fall M. Intravesical bacillus Calmette-Guerin and dimethyl sulfoxide for treatment of classic and nonulcer interstitial cystitis: a prospective, randomized double-blind study. J Urol 2000;164: 1912,5; discussion 1915–6. (Level II-3)

61. Moldwin RM, Evans RJ, Stanford EJ, Rosenberg MT. Rational approaches to the treatment of patients with interstitial cystitis. Urology 2007;69:73–81. (Level III)

62. Maher CF, Carey MP, Dwyer PL, Schluter PL. Percutaneous sacral nerve root neuromodulation for intractable interstitial cystitis. J Urol 2001;165:884–6. (Level III)

63. Peters KM, Konstandt D. Sacral neuromodulation decreases narcotic requirements in refractory interstitial cystitis. BJU Int 2004;93:777–9. (Level III)

64. Foster DC, Kotok MB, Huang LS, Watts A, Oakes D, Howard FM, et al. Oral desipramine and topical lidocaine for vulvodynia: a randomized controlled trial. Obstet Gynecol 2010;116:583–93. (Level I)

65. Dede M, Yenen MC, Yilmaz A, Baser I. Successful treatment of persistent vulvodynia with submucous infiltration of betamethasone and lidocaine. Eur J Obstet Gynecol Reprod Biol 2006;124:258–9. (Level III—letter)

66. Rapkin AJ, McDonald JS, Morgan M. Multilevel local anesthetic nerve blockade for the treatment of vulvar vestibulitis syndrome. Am J Obstet Gynecol 2008;198:41.e1–41.e5. (Level III)

67. Bergeron S, Binik YM, Khalife S, Pagidas K, Glazer HI, Meana M, et al. A randomized comparison of group cognitive--behavioral therapy, surface electromyographic biofeedback, and vestibulectomy in the treatment of dyspareunia resulting from vulvar vestibulitis. Pain 2001;91:297–306. (Level I)

68. Tommola P, Unkila-Kallio L, Paavonen J. Surgical treatment of vulvar vestibulitis: a review. Acta Obstet Gynecol Scand 2010;89:1385–95. (Level III)

69. Haefner HK. Critique of new gynecologic surgical procedures: surgery for vulvar vestibulitis. Clin Obstet Gynecol 2000;43:689–700. (Level III)

70. Drossman DA, Dumitrascu DL. Rome III: New standard for functional gastrointestinal disorders. J Gastrointestin Liver Dis 2006;15:237–41. (Level III)

71. Mayer EA. Clinical practice. Irritable bowel syndrome. N Engl J Med 2008; 358:1692–9. (Level III)

72. Rahimi R, Nikfar S, Rezaie A, Abdollahi M. Efficacy of tricyclic antidepressants in irritable bowel syndrome: a meta-analysis. World J Gastroenterol 2009;15:1548–53. (Meta-analysis)

73. Affaitati G, Fabrizio A, Savini A, Lerza R, Tafuri E, Constantini R, et al. A randomized, controlled study comparing a lidocaine patch, a placebo patch, and anesthetic injection for treatment of trigger points in patients with myofascial pain syndrome: evaluation of pain and somatic pain thresholds. Clin Ther 2009;31:705–20. (Level I)

74. Butrick CW. Pelvic floor hypertonic disorders: identification and management. Obstet Gynecol Clin North Am 2009;36:707–22. (Level III)

75. FitzGerald MP, Anderson RU, Potts J, Payne CK, Peters KM, Clemens JQ, et al. Randomized multicenter feasibility trial of myofascial physical therapy for the treatment of urological chronic pelvic pain syndromes. Urological Pelvic Pain Collaborative Research Network. J Urol 2009;182:570–80. (Level I)

76. Abbott JA, Jarvis SK, Lyons SD, Thomson A, Vancaille TG. Botulinum toxin type A for chronic pain and pelvic floor spasm in women: a randomized controlled trial. Obstet Gynecol 2006;108:915–23. (Level I)

77. Crofford LJ. Pain management in fibromyalgia. Curr Opin Rheumatol 2008; 20:246–50. (Level III)

78. Hauser W, Bernardy K, Uceyler N, Sommer C. Treatment of fibromyalgia syndrome with antidepressants: a meta-analysis. JAMA 2009;301:198–209. (Meta-analysis)

79. Baker PK. Musculoskeletal origins of chronic pelvic pain. Diagnosis and treatment. Obstet Gynecol Clin North Am 1993;20:719–42. (Level III)

80. O'Connor AB, Dworkin RH. Treatment of neuropathic pain: an overview of recent guidelines. Am J Med 2009;122:S22–32. (Level III)

81. Fishbain DA, Cole B, Lewis J, Rosomoff HL, Rosomoff RS. What percentage of chronic nonmalignant pain patients exposed to chronic opioid analgesic therapy develop abuse/addiction and/or aberrant drug-related behaviors? A structured evidence-based review. Pain Med 2008;9:444–59. (Level III)

82. Hojsted J, Sjorgen P. Addiction to opioids in chronic pain patients: a literature review. Eur J Pain 2007;11:490–518. (Level III)

83. Engel CC Jr, Walker EA, Engel AL, Bullis J, Armstrong A. A randomized, double-blind crossover trial of sertraline in women with chronic pelvic pain. J Psychosom Res 1998;44:203–7. (Level II-3)

84. Sator-Katzenschlager SM, Scharbert G, Kress HG, Frickey N, Ellend A, Gleiss A, et al. Chronic pelvic pain treated with gabapentin and amitriptyline: a randomized controlled pilot study. Wien Klin Wochenschr 2005;117:761–8. (Level I)

85. Slocumb JC. Chronic somatic, myofascial, and neurogenic abdominal pelvic pain. Clin Obstet Gynecol 1990;33:145–53. (Level III)

86. Langford CF, Udvari Nagy S, Ghoniem GM. Levator ani trigger point injections: an underutilized treatment for chronic pelvic pain. Neurourol Urodyn 2007;26:59–62. (Level III)

87. Romito S, Bottanelli M, Pellegrini M, Vicentini S, Rizzuto N, Bertolasi L. Botulinum toxin for the treatment of genital pain syndromes. Gynecol Obstet Invest 2004;58:164–7. (Level III)

88. Thomson AJ, Jarvis SK, Lenart M, Abbott JA, Vancaillie TG. The use of botulinum toxin type A (BOTOX) as treatment for intractable chronic pelvic pain associated with spasm of the levator ani muscles. BJOG 2005;112:247–9. (Level III)

89. Lamvu G, Tu F, As-Sanie S, Zolnoun D, Steege JF. The role of laparoscopy in the diagnosis and treatment of conditions associated with chronic pelvic pain. Obstet Gynecol Clin North Am 2004;31:619–30, x. (Level III)

90. Peters AA, van Dorst E, Jellis B, van Zuuren E, Hermans J, Trimbos JB. A randomized clinical trial to compare two different approaches in women with chronic pelvic pain. Obstet Gynecol 1991;77:740–4. (Level I)

91. Daniels J, Gray R, Hills RK, Latthe P, Buckley L, Gupta J, et al. Laparoscopic uterosacral nerve ablation for alleviating chronic pelvic pain: a randomized controlled trial. LUNA Trial Collaboration. JAMA 2009;302:955–61. (Level I)

92. Candiani GB, Fedele L, Vercellini P, Bianchi S, Di Nola G. Presacral neurectomy for the treatment of pelvic pain associated with endometriosis: a controlled study. Am J Obstet Gynecol 1992;167:100–3. (Level I)

93. Tjaden B, Schlaff WD, Kimball A, Rock JA. The efficacy of presacral neurectomy for the relief of midline dysmenorrhea. Obstet Gynecol 1990;76:89–91. (Level III)

94. Zullo F, Palomba S, Zupi E, Russo T, Morelli M, Cappiello F, et al. Effectiveness of presacral neurectomy in women with severe dysmenorrhea caused by endometriosis who were treated with laparoscopic conservative surgery: a 1-year prospective randomized double-blind controlled trial. Am J Obstet Gynecol 2003;189:5–10. (Level I)

95. Vercellini P, Vigano P, Somigliana E, Abbiati A, Barbara G, Fedele L. Medical, surgical and alternative treatments for chronic pelvic pain in women: a descriptive review. Gynecol Endocrinol 2009;25:208–21. (Level III)

96. Latthe PM, Proctor ML, Farquhar CM, Johnson N, Khan KS. Surgical interruption of pelvic nerve pathways in dysmenorrhea: a systematic review of effectiveness. Acta Obstet Gynecol Scand 2007;86:4–15. (Meta-analysis)

97. Carlson KJ, Miller BA, Fowler FJ Jr. The Maine women's health study: II. Outcomes of nonsurgical management of leiomyomas, abnormal bleeding, and chronic pelvic pain. Obstet Gynecol 1994;83:566–72. (Level II-3)

98. Hillis SD, Marchbanks PA, Peterson HB. The effectiveness of hysterectomy for chronic pelvic pain. Obstet Gynecol 1995;86:941–5. (Level II-3)

99. O'Mathúna DP. Herb-drug interactions. Altern Med Alert 2003;6:37–43. (Level III)

100. Fugh-Berman A, Kronenberg F. Complementary and alternative medicine (CAM) in reproductive-age women: a review of randomized controlled trials. Reprod Toxicol 2003;17:137–52. (Level III)

101. Teets RY, Dahmer S, Scott E. Integrative medicine approach to chronic pain. Prim Care 2010;37:407–21. (Level III)

102. Posadzki P, Ernst E. Yoga for low back pain: a systematic review of randomized clinical trials. Clin Rheumatol 2011;30:1257–62. (Level III)

103. Tan G, Craine MH, Bair MJ, Garcia MK, Giordano J, Jensen MP, et al. Efficacy of selected complementary and alternative medicine interventions for chronic pain. J Rehabil Res Dev 2007;44:195–222. (Level III)

104. Cho SH, Hwang EW. Acupuncture for primary dysmenorrhoea: a systematic review. BJOG 2010;117:509–21. (Level III)

105. Proctor M, Farquhar C, Stones W, He L, Zhu X, Brown J. Transcutaneous electrical nerve stimulation for primary dysmenorrhoea. Cochrane Database of Systematic Reviews 2002, Issue 1. Art. No.: CD002123. DOI: 10.1002/14651858.CD002123; 10.1002/14651858.CD002123. (Meta-analysis)

106. Murina F, Bianco V, Radici G, Felice R, Di Martino M, Nicolini U. Transcutaneous electrical nerve stimulation to treat vestibulodynia: a randomised controlled trial. BJOG 2008;115:1165–70. (Level I)

107. Abram SE, Haddox JD. The pain clinic manual. 2nd ed. Philadelphia (PA): Lippincott Williams and Wilkins; 2000. (Level III)

108. Vermani E, Mittal R, Weeks A. Pelvic girdle pain and low back pain in pregnancy: a review. Pain Pract 2009;10:60–71. (Level III)

109. Sax TW, Rosenbaum RB. Neuromuscular disorders in pregnancy. Muscle Nerve 2006;34:559–71. (Level III)

110. Chung CS, Myrianthopoulos NC. Factors affecting risks of congenital malformations. I. Analysis of epidemiologic factors in congenital malformations. Report from the Collaborative Perinatal Project. Birth Defects Orig Artic Ser 1975;11:1–22. (Level II-3)

111. Heinonen OP, Shapiro S, Slone D. Birth defects and drugs in pregnancy. Littleton, Mass.: Publishing Sciences Group; 1977. (Level III)

112. Wisner KL, Gelenberg AJ, Leonard H, Zarin D, Frank E. Pharmacologic treatment of depression during pregnancy. JAMA 1999;282:1264–9. (Level III)

113. Tuccori M, Montagnani S, Testi A, Ruggiero E, Mantarro S, Scollo C, et al. Use of selective serotonin reuptake inhibitors during pregnancy and risk of major and cardiovascular malformations: an update. Postgrad Med 2010;122:49–65. (Level III)

114. Bar-Oz B, Einarson T, Einarson A, Boskovic R, O'Brien L, Malm H, et al. Paroxetine and congenital malformations: meta-analysis and consideration of potential confounding factors. Clin Ther 2007;29:918–26. (Meta-analysis)

115. Chambers CD, Johnson KA, Dick LM, Felix RJ, Jones KL. Birth outcomes in pregnant women taking fluoxetine. N Engl J Med 1996;335:1010–5. (Level II-2)

116. Chambers CD, Hernandez-Diaz S, Van Marter LJ, Werler MM, Louik C, Jones KL, et al. Selective serotonin-reuptake inhibitors and risk of persistent pulmonary hypertension of the newborn. N Engl J Med 2006;354:579–87. (Level II-2)

117. Rathmell JP, Viscomi CM, Ashburn MA. Management of nonobstetric pain during pregnancy and lactation. Anesth Analg 1997;85:1074–87. (Level III)

118. Dowswell T, Bedwell C, Lavender T, Neilson James P. Transcutaneous electrical nerve stimulation (TENS) for pain relief in labour. Cochrane Database of Systematic Reviews 2009, Issue 2. Art. No.: CD007214. DOI: 10.1002/14651858.CD007214.pub2; 10.1002/14651858.CD007214.pub2. (Meta-analysis)

119. Ee CC, Manheimer E, Pirotta MV, White AR. Acupuncture for pelvic and back pain in pregnancy: a systematic review. Am J Obstet Gynecol 2008;198:254–9. (Level III)

120. Schecter WP, Farmer D, Horn JK, Pietrocola DM, Wallace A. Special considerations in perioperative pain management: audiovisual distraction, geriatrics, pediatrics, and pregnancy. J Am Coll Surg 2005;201:612–8. (Level III)

121. Abouleish E, Rawal N, Rashad MN. The addition of 0.2 mg subarachnoid morphine to hyperbaric bupivacaine for cesarean delivery: a prospective study of 856 cases. Reg Anesth 1991;16:137–40. (Level III)

122. Girgin NK, Gurbet A, Turker G, Aksu H, Gulhan N. Intrathecal morphine in anesthesia for cesarean delivery: dose-response relationship for combinations of low-dose intrathecal morphine and spinal bupivacaine. J Clin Anesth 2008;20:180–5. (Level I)

123. Abboud TK, Dror A, Mosaad P, Zhu J, Mantilla M, Swart F, et al. Mini-dose intrathecal morphine for the relief of post-cesarean section pain: safety, efficacy, and ventilatory responses to carbon dioxide. Anesth Analg 1988;67:137–43. (Level I)

124. Angle P, Walsh V. Pain relief after cesarean section. Tech Reg Anesth Pain Manag 2001;5:36–40. (Level III)

125. Liu SS, Wu CL. The effect of analgesic technique on postoperative patient-reported outcomes including analgesia: a systematic review. Anesth Analg 2007;105:789–808. (Level III)

126. Hutchison RW, Hae Chon E, Tucker WF, Gilder R, Moss J, Daniel P. A comparison of a Fentanyl, Morphine, and Hydromorphone patient-controlled intravenous delivery for acute postoperative analgesia: a multicenter study of opioid-induced adverse reactions. Hosp Pharm 2006;41:659–63. (Level II-3)

127. Rapp SE, Egan KJ, Ross BK, Wild LM, Terman GW, Ching JM. A multidimensional comparison of morphine and hydromorphone patient-controlled analgesia. Anesth Analg 1996;82:1043–8. (Level I)

128. Moore RA, Derry S, McQuay Henry J. Single dose oral dexibupro-
fen [S(+)-ibuprofen] for acute postoperative pain in adults. Cochrane
Database of Systematic Reviews 2009, Issue 3. Art. No.: CD007550. DOI:
10.1002/14651858.CD007550.pub2; 10.1002/14651858.CD007550.pub2.
(Level III)

129. Buck L, Varras MN, Miskry T, Ruston J, Magos A. Intraperitoneal bupivacaine for the reduction of postoperative pain following operative laparoscopy: a pilot study and review of the literature. J Obstet Gynaecol
2004;24:448–51. (Level III)

130. Baig MK, Zmora O, Derdemezi J, Weiss EG, Nogueras JJ, Wexner SD. Use of
the ON-Q pain management system is associated with decreased postoperative analgesic requirement: double blind randomized placebo pilot study. J Am
Coll Surg 2006;202:297–305. (Level I)

131. Stevenson DG, Bramson JS. Hospice care in the nursing home setting: a
review of the literature. J Pain Symptom Manage 2009;38:440–51. (Level III)

132. Savage SR. Management of opioid medications in patients with chronic pain
and risk of substance misuse. Curr Psychiatr Rep 2009;11:377–84. (Level III)

Studies were reviewed and evaluated for quality according to the
method outlined by the U.S. Preventive Services Task Force:

I   Evidence obtained from at least one properly designed randomized controlled trial.

II-1 Evidence obtained from well-designed controlled trials without
randomization.

II-2 Evidence obtained from well-designed cohort or case–control
analytic studies, preferably from more than one center or
research group.

II-3 Evidence obtained from multiple time series with or without
the intervention. Dramatic results in uncontrolled experiments
also could be regarded as this type of evidence.

III Opinions of respected authorities, based on clinical experience,
descriptive studies, or reports of expert committees.

Answers

1. B, 2. C, 3. A, 4. B, 5. D, 6. C, 7. D, 8. B, 9. B, 10. B, 11. C, 12. C, 13. A, 14. A,
15. B, 16. D, 17. B, 18. B, 19. C, 20. C

Index

152

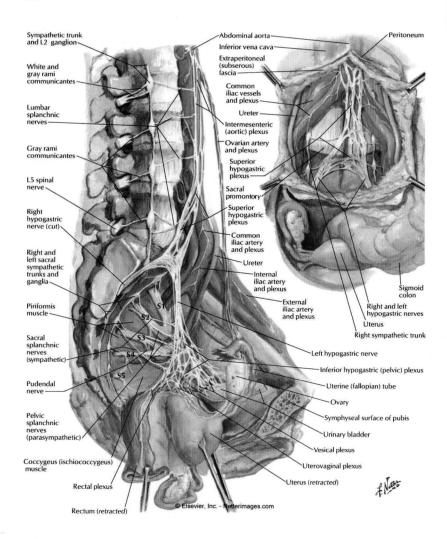

Sympathetic trunk and L2 ganglion

White and gray rami communicantes

Lumbar splanchnic nerves

Gray rami communicantes

L5 spinal nerve

Right hypogastric nerve (*cut*)

Right and left sacral sympathetic trunks and ganglia

Piriformis muscle

Sacral splanchnic nerves (sympathetic)

Pudendal nerve

Pelvic splanchnic nerves (parasympathetic)

Coccygeus (ischiococcygeus) muscle

Rectal plexus

Rectum (*retracted*)

Abdominal aorta

Inferior vena cava

Extraperitoneal (subserous) fascia

Common iliac vessels and plexus

Ureter

Intermesenteric (aortic) plexus

Ovarian artery and plexus

Superior hypogastric plexus

Sacral promontory

Superior hypogastric plexus

Common iliac artery and plexus

Ureter

Internal iliac artery and plexus

External iliac artery and plexus

S1

S2

S3

S4

S5

Peritoneum

Sigmoid colon

Right and left hypogastric nerves

Uterus

Right sympathetic trunk

Left hypogastric nerve

Inferior hypogastric (pelvic) plexus

Uterine (fallopian) tube

Ovary

Symphyseal surface of pubis

Urinary bladder

Vesical plexus

Uterovaginal plexus

Uterus (*retracted*)

Fig. 1. Pelvic cavity: sacral and thoracolumbar autonomic nerves. (Frank H. Netter. Atlas of human anatomy. 4th ed. Philadelphia [PA]: Saunders; 2006. p. 412. Netter illustration from www.netterimages.com. © Elsevier, Inc. All rights reserved.)

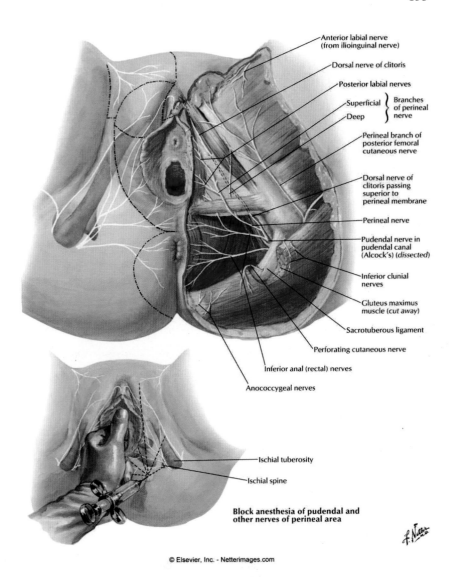

Anterior labial nerve
(from ilioinguinal nerve)

Dorsal nerve of clitoris

Posterior labial nerves

Superficial } Branches
Deep } of perineal nerve

Perineal branch of posterior femoral cutaneous nerve

Dorsal nerve of clitoris passing superior to perineal membrane

Perineal nerve

Pudendal nerve in pudendal canal (Alcock's) (*dissected*)

Inferior clunial nerves

Gluteus maximus muscle (*cut away*)

Sacrotuberous ligament

Perforating cutaneous nerve

Inferior anal (rectal) nerves

Anococcygeal nerves

Ischial tuberosity

Ischial spine

Block anesthesia of pudendal and other nerves of perineal area

Fig. 2. Nerves of perineum and external genitalia. (Frank H. Netter. Atlas of human anatomy. 4th ed. Philadelphia [PA]: Saunders; 2006. p. 413. Netter illustration from www.netterimages.com. © Elsevier, Inc. All rights reserved.)

154

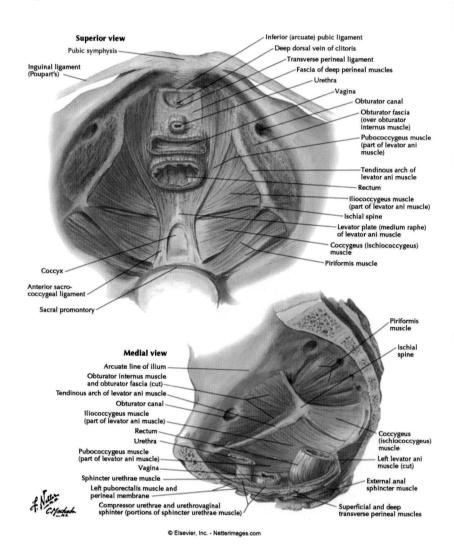

Fig. 5. Muscles of the pelvic floor and perineum. (Frank H. Netter. Atlas of human anatomy. 4th ed. Philadelphia [PA]: Saunders; 2006. p. 356. Netter illustration from www.netterimages.com. © Elsevier, Inc. All rights reserved.)

Forthcoming Titles

Each monograph in *Clinical Updates in Women's Health Care* is an overview of a topic of importance to obstetrician–gynecologists in practice. Upcoming titles include:

- Addiction and Substance Abuse
- Asthma

If not previously completed, earn 5 CME credits for back issues of *Clinical Updates in Women's Health Care*. Listed are recent titles. For a complete list of titles, visit www.clinicalupdates.org:

- *Anorectal Disorders* (Volume IX, Number 1, January 2010)
- *Continuing Care for Women With Breast Cancer* (Volume IX, Number 2, April 2010)
- *Occupational Diseases and Injuries* (Volume IX, Number 3, July 2010)
- *Perioperative Considerations for Coexisting Medical Conditions* (Volume IX, Number 4, October 2010)
- *Multiple Sclerosis* (Volume IX, Number 5, November 2010)
- *Renal Disease* (Volume X, Number 1, January 2011)
- *Dyslipidemia* (Volume X, Number 2, April 2011)
- *Heart Disease* (Volume X, Number 3, July 2011)
- *Complementary and Alternative Medicine* (Volume X, Number 4, October 2011)

You can sign up for a 1-year subscription to *Clinical Updates in Women's Health Care* at the rate of $59 for College members ($105 nonmembers). Individual copies also can be purchased for $25 ($35 nonmembers). You can subscribe by calling (800) 762-2264 or online at sales.acog.org. Online access is available to subscribers at www.clinicalupdates.org.

The Editorial Board welcomes comments and suggestions for topics. Please contact the Editorial Board in care of College Publications (publication@acog.org).

CLINICAL UPDATES
IN WOMEN'S HEALTH CARE

Pain Management

Volume X, Number 5, November 2011

Test Your Clinical Skills—and Earn CME Credits

ACCME Accreditation

The American College of Obstetricians and Gynecologists is accredited by the Accreditation Council for Continuing Medical Education (ACCME) to provide continuing medical education for physicians.

AMA PRA Category 1 Credit™ and College Cognate Credit

The American College of Obstetricians and Gynecologists designates this educational activity for a maximum of 5 AMA PRA Category 1 Credit(s)™ or up to a maximum of 5 Category 1 College Cognate Credit(s). Physicians should only claim credit commensurate with the extent of their participation in the activity.

Credit for *Clinical Updates in Women's Health Care: Pain Management,* Volume X, Number 5, November 2011, is initially available through December 2014. During that year, the unit will be reevaluated. If the content remains current, credit is extended for an additional 3 years.

Actual time spent completing this activity (you may record up to 5 hours):_____.

To obtain credits, complete and return this answer sheet to the address shown below (only original answer sheets will be accepted for credit) or submit your answers online at www.clinicalupdates.org:

1. _____	8. _____	15. _____
2. _____	9. _____	16. _____
3. _____	10. _____	17. _____
4. _____	11. _____	18. _____
5. _____	12. _____	19. _____
6. _____	13. _____	20. _____
7. _____	14. _____	

ACOG ID Number __ __ __ __ __ __ __ __ __ __

Name _____

Address_____

City/State/Zip _____

The American College of Obstetricians and Gynecologists
Educational Development and Testing
409 12th Street, SW
PO Box 96920
Washington, DC 20090-6920

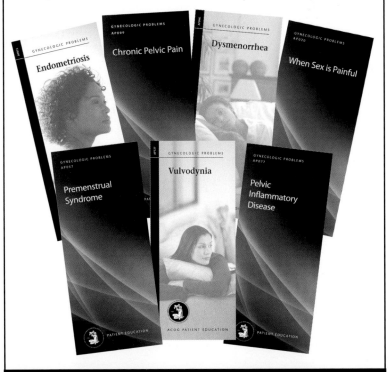

Powerful Communication Skills:

How to Communicate with Confidence, Clarity and Credibility

Written by Colleen McKenna

Edited by National Press Publications

NATIONAL PRESS PUBLICATIONS

A Division of Rockhurst College Continuing Education Center, Inc.

6901 West 63rd St., P.O. Box 2949, Shawnee Mission, KS 66201-1349

1-800-258-7248 • 1-913-432-7757

National Press Publications endorses non-sexist language. However, in an effort to make this handbook clear, consistent and easy to read, we've used "he" throughout the odd-numbered chapters when referring to both males and females, and we've used "she" throughout the even-numbered chapters when referring to both males and females. The copy is not intended to be sexist.

Powerful Communication Skills: How to Communicate
with Confidence, Clarity and Credibility
Published by National Press Publications, Inc.
Copyright 1997, National Press Publications, Inc.
A Division of Rockhurst College Continuing Education Center, Inc.

Printed in the United States of America

1 2 3 4 5 6 7 8 9 10

ISBN 1-55852-215-8